D0485601

The
NEWBORN
HANDBOOK

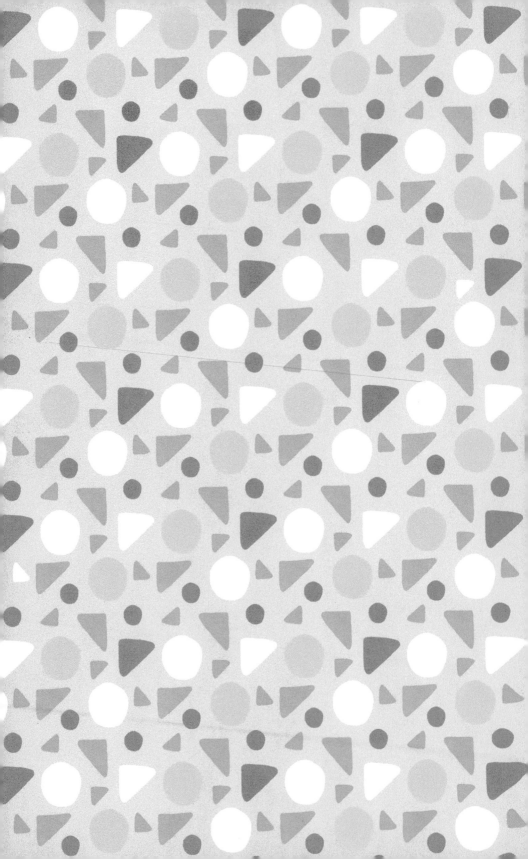

The
NEWBORN
HANDBOOK

Your Guide to Bringing Home Baby

From
0 through
3 Months

Dr. Smita Malhotra, MD
Illustrated by Sarah Smart

**ROCKRIDGE
PRESS**

For general information on our other products and services or to obtain technical support, please contact our Customer Care Department within the United States at (866) 744-2665, or outside the United States at (510) 253-0500.

Interior and Cover Designer: Jill Lee
Art Producer: Karen Williams
Editor: Kelly Koester
Production Editor: Nora Milman

Illustration © 2020 Sarah Smart.

ISBN: Print 978-1-64739-631-2 | eBook 978-1-64739-632-9

R0

To my daughters,
Sahana and Simran, who
allow me to be imperfect
and love me anyway.
I will always belong to you.

To my husband, Gil,
without whose support
this book could not have
been written.
I am a better mother
with you by my side.

CONTENTS

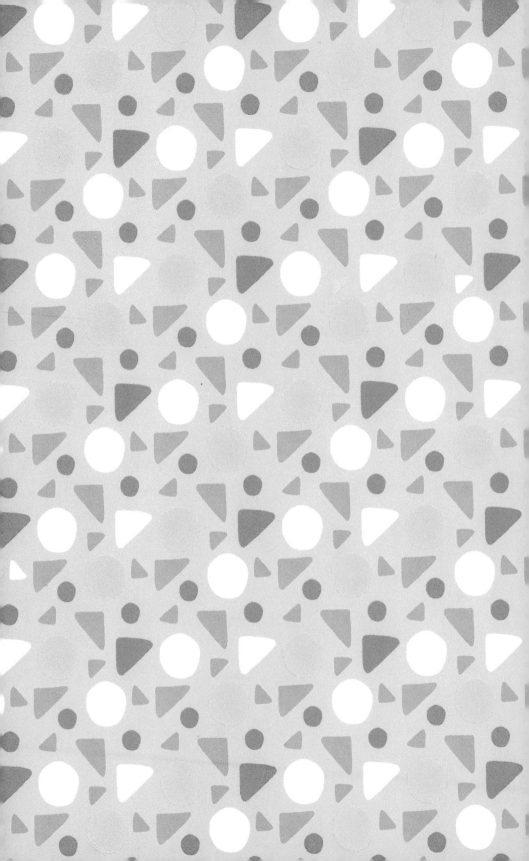

INTRODUCTION

Becoming a parent transformed me as a pediatrician. For more than a decade, I have cared for thousands of children and guided parents through the first few months with a newborn. But it was only after my own children were born that I was able to give medical advice with a different kind of understanding, one that comes from the shared experience of new parenthood.

I empathize with the pain and frustration some mothers experienced. Instructions to feed a newborn every two to three hours come with the realization that parents did not necessarily get any rest in between those hours. Telling a parent that their child had a cold comes with the understanding that despite the benign diagnosis, that parent will still stay up all night watching their child's chest to make sure she is breathing.

The medical advice remained the same. But I understood its impact on my patients and their parents in a much deeper way.

The guidance in this book is not solely advice from a pediatrician; it is wrapped in lessons learned beyond medical school and residency. It is intended to lead you gently through caring for a newborn in the first three months—the months that can be both exhilarating and nerve-racking at the same time. No matter how your baby came into your life, this book is for all parents and caregivers.

Although I may someday stop practicing pediatrics, I will never stop being a parent because being a parent is a commitment we make for a lifetime. And that lifetime is about to begin for you.

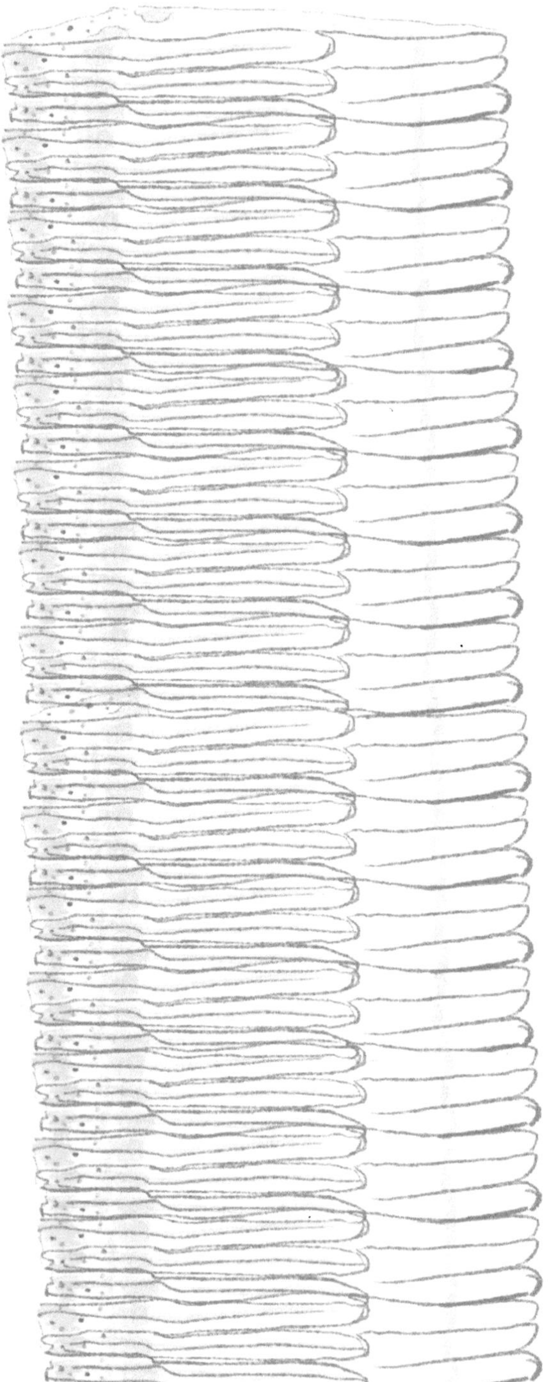

PART ONE

Before Your Baby's Arrival

You are about to embark on one of the most challenging, vulnerable, and fulfilling journeys of your life. One that will open hidden parts of your heart. And while you will never be fully prepared for the unexpected turns of parenthood, there are steps you can take in advance to prepare for bringing your newborn home.

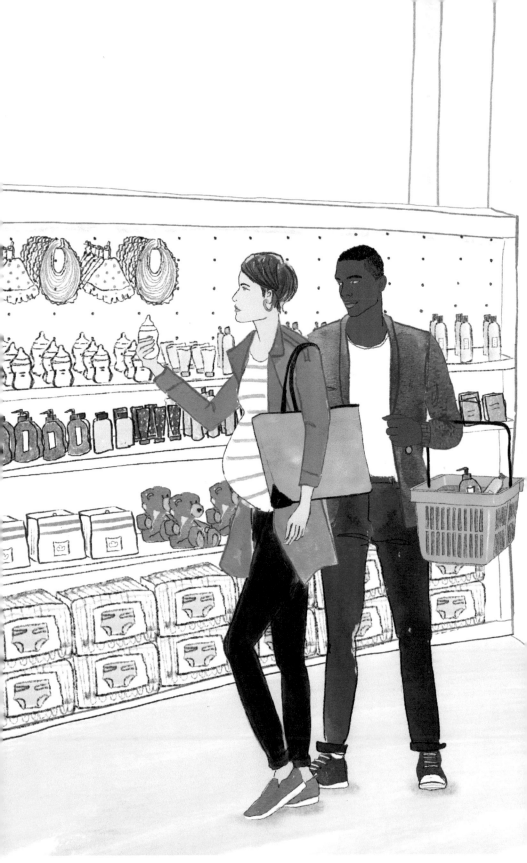

CHAPTER
1

Getting Your Home Ready for Baby

• •

The first few months with a newborn are a whirlwind of feeding and sleep deprivation, so it is helpful to prepare your home to minimize any extra stress in this initial period. With a little planning, you will be able to concentrate on your most important goal—bonding with your baby!

Sleeping Supplies

One of the main needs all newborns share is sleep. Spending some time preparing where and how your baby will sleep is important because this will help keep your newborn safe. Additionally, setting up baby's sleep space will help you settle into a routine once she comes home.

Where Should Your Baby Sleep?

One of the most fun tasks for many expecting parents is decorating their newborn's nursery. But keep in mind that your newborn likely won't be sleeping in this space for several months. The American Academy of Pediatrics (AAP) recommends that for at least the first six months (preferably up to one year), babies should sleep in the same room as their parents, on their backs on a separate surface. Sharing a bed with your baby is not recommended. If your baby rolls onto their stomach or side when they are sleeping, you can reposition him, and having baby in your room helps with this. Even if he doesn't sleep in that new nursery right away, you can always use it as a playroom and admire your design skills!

What Should Your Baby Sleep In?

A safe sleep environment for your newborn should include a firm surface, such as a crib or a bassinet with a tight-fitting sheet. Make sure that the crib or bassinet you intend to use meets current safety standards and has not been recalled. Keep the crib away from windows and any cords that can be pulled or that might pose strangulation hazards as your baby becomes mobile. While newborn blankets, pillows, and stuffed animals are absolutely adorable, it is important not to keep these in the crib when your newborn is sleeping. You can always use them during playtime or to create cute photos to share with your loved ones.

Feeding Supplies

Every family has different needs and responsibilities. Therefore, the decision to formula feed or breastfeed is personal to each family. If you are trying to decide what is best for yours, read Deciding to Breastfeed (or Not!) on page 9. Regardless of how you choose to feed your baby, here are some supplies that you will need:

- Bibs
- Bottle brushes
- Bottles
- Burp cloths

Breastfeeding Supplies

If you are a mother who is choosing to breastfeed, these are some items that will make feedings easier:

- **Breast milk storage bags.** If you are pumping, you will need bags to store the milk. Purchase bags that are intended for freezing so that you can store milk for future months, which will be helpful if you go back to work. Store the bags flat in the freezer so they'll take up less space and thaw faster.

- **Breast pump.** Invest in a good breast pump. Life with a newborn can be unpredictable, and it is helpful to have stored breast milk for unexpected situations when you may need to be away from baby. If you plan to return to work after your baby is born, start pumping your milk and storing it early so that you have a supply built up when maternity leave ends.

- **Nipple cream.** Although breastfeeding is a great opportunity to bond with your newborn, the pain from cracked nipples can make feeding an uncomfortable experience. The right nipple cream will make all the difference. Lanolin is safe to use on intact skin and nipples, and it will not harm your baby. If you or your baby have any discomfort with the cream, please consult your pediatrician.

- **Nursing bras or tanks.** Most nursing bras have drop-down cups so you can conveniently feed your newborn. Purchase a size up when you are nursing because your breasts will fill with milk. Nursing tanks are another great option if you prefer belly coverage. In general, it is good to have at least three nursing bras or tanks so that even if one is in the wash, you still have an extra one on hand in case something happens to the one you're wearing (such as baby spit-up).

- **Nursing pads.** Your breasts are going to leak. And they may leak in public! Nursing pads are lifesavers for avoiding those potentially embarrassing situations.

- **Nursing pillows.** When you spend your days breastfeeding and being sleep-deprived, you will welcome any opportunity for rest. The right nursing pillow helps keep your baby in a comfortable position for nursing and gives your arms a much-needed break.

Formula Supplies

If you are a parent who is choosing to feed with formula, here are some supplies you may need:

- **Bottle warmer.** For those middle-of-the-night feedings when you want to warm the bottle quickly, a bottle warmer will help you and your baby get back to sleep faster. Although this is not a must-have item, it certainly makes life easier, and over time the little time-savers add up!

- **Bottles and bottle nipples.** There are several types of bottles and nipples. Bottle nipples come in different levels based on how a newborn is feeding. Instead of investing in several bottles and nipples that are all the same type, buy a few different kinds until you learn which type works best for your baby.

- **Formula mixer.** Much like a coffee machine, a formula mixer can make enough formula for an entire day at the right temperature. Like the bottle warmer, this is not a must-have item, but it's definitely something to consider, especially if you will not have a lot of help in the first few months.

- **Formula.** The good news is that all formulas marketed in the United States must meet basic nutrient requirements, so the brand you choose is less important than you might think. Since every baby is different, pick a formula that your newborn tolerates well. This may take some trial and error. It is generally recommended to give your baby about a week to adjust to a new formula. However, if your baby has excessive fussiness, gas, loose stools, or blood in the stools, please consult your pediatrician.

DECIDING TO BREASTFEED (OR NOT!)

Breastfeeding has many benefits. Breast milk provides the ideal amount of nutrients for babies, and it contains antibodies that help protect newborns from respiratory infections and diarrhea.

However, breastfeeding is not for everyone. Many parents choose not to breastfeed, and this is okay.

I had every intention of breastfeeding my children, but because of issues with milk production, things did not go as planned. My struggles with breastfeeding early in my parenting journey gave me a gift that I have come back to many times in my years of parenthood: the gift of self-compassion.

In parenting, as in life, things don't always work out how we want them to. No one will ask your adult child if they were breastfed or formula-fed.

If you are a mother who is hoping to breastfeed and have a plan for how you will feed your baby (as the hospital will ask you), understand that plans can change. And if they do, treat yourself with compassion. Sometimes our changing hormones after delivery can exacerbate our feelings and cause us to be especially hard on ourselves. Remember that how you choose to safely feed your baby is not a reflection on your ability as a parent.

There is no room for judgment in parenting, so why judge yourself?

Too Soon for Babyproofing?

When your baby arrives, there will be so much going on that babyproofing your home will be at the bottom of your list, but it is not too soon to start babyproofing. While a newborn will not be crawling around the house, there are things you should address in your home that could pose a risk as your baby grows.

Secure any unstable furniture (such as TV stands that could fall over) and any rugs that may be easy for you to slip on while holding your baby. Make sure that the smoke detectors in your home are installed and function properly. If your home was built before 1978, get your home checked for lead-based paint. The dust from peeling lead-based paint can be harmful to the development of a growing child.

As your baby grows and starts crawling, you will want to cover electrical outlets and install baby gates on your stairs. You should move dangerous household items away from your baby's reach and start padding sharp furniture edges.

Remember that it's easier to get these things ready now before you join the ranks of sleep-deprived parents everywhere!

Keeping Your Newborn Safe

Almost every parent has felt a sense of nervousness when they hold their newborn for the first time. These little beings may look fragile, but they are remarkably resilient. In this section, we will discuss some ways to help keep your newborn as safe as possible and put your mind at ease.

Preventing Sudden Infant Death Syndrome

According to the AAP, about 3,500 otherwise healthy babies die in their sleep before their first birthday each year in the United States. This is known as sudden infant death syndrome (SIDS). Although the cause of SIDS is not known, research has shown that there are several things you can do to greatly reduce this risk.

PUT YOUR BABY TO SLEEP ON THEIR BACK, EVEN DURING NAPS.

Until one year of age, babies should be put to sleep on their back at night and during naps. Babies who fall asleep in devices such as car seats, strollers, or swings should be moved to a flat and firm surface.

PUT YOUR BABY TO SLEEP ON A FLAT AND FIRM SURFACE, SUCH AS A CRIB OR BASSINET.

Make sure that the crib or bassinet that you buy has not been recalled and that the hardware is intact. You will also want to use a tight-fitting sheet. If you swaddle your newborn, swaddling should stop when your baby starts rolling over.

KEEP BLANKETS, PILLOWS, STUFFED ANIMALS, AND SOFT BEDDING AWAY FROM THE CRIB.

These items can increase the risk of suffocation. Although these are popular gifts for baby showers, save them for playtime instead of nap and sleep time.

YOU CAN SHARE A ROOM WITH YOUR BABY UNTIL SHE IS ONE YEAR OLD, BUT YOU SHOULD SLEEP ON DIFFERENT SURFACES.

Research has shown that sharing a room with your baby can decrease the risk of SIDS by as much as 50 percent. However, the AAP recommends against sharing a bed with your baby because of the risk of a parent rolling over onto the baby or the baby suffocating in the sheets.

STAY AWAY FROM SMOKING.

If you are a smoker, make every attempt to quit, for your own health and for your baby's. In addition, keep your baby away from areas where people are or have been smoking. Maintaining a smoke-free environment for your child can reduce the risk of SIDS.

KEEP YOUR BABY COOL.

In the winter months, parents want to layer their baby in warm clothes, but keeping your baby too warm can increase the risk of SIDS. When the temperature drops, dress your baby in only one extra layer than what feels comfortable for you. For instance, if you are fine in a single layer, your baby needs no more than two layers.

OFFER YOUR BABY A PACIFIER.

The use of a pacifier during naps and sleep can help decrease the risk of SIDS. However, if you are breastfeeding, it is recommended to wait for at least 4 weeks, or until breastfeeding has been established, to introduce a pacifier. Keep in mind not all babies will like a pacifier, and this is okay. Also, do not use pacifiers that come in two pieces or that are attached to other objects because of the increased risk of choking.

A Note on Bed-Sharing

I do not recommend bed-sharing. Your baby should sleep in their own bed, in the same room as you. However, I understand that amid being overwhelmed and tired, parents sometimes fall asleep next to their baby. If you think you may fall asleep while feeding, feed your baby on the bed rather than on the sofa or in a chair. Make sure there are no pillows, sheets, or blankets near your baby as they pose a risk of suffocation. When you wake up, remember to move your baby to their own bed. Please do not bed-share if your baby was born premature, if you are a smoker, if you have consumed alcohol, or if you have used any illicit substances or medications that can cause impairment.

Must-Have Item: Car Seat

One item you absolutely must have before your newborn arrives is a car seat. You won't be able to leave the hospital without one!

There are four types of car seats: rear-facing, convertible, forward-facing, and booster seats.

For newborns, you'll want to get a rear-facing car seat or a convertible car seat that can be converted to forward-facing as your baby grows. Newborns should be rear-facing until they are at least 2 years of age and they reach the highest height and/or weight allowed by the manufacturer of your seat.

The seat of a rear-facing car seat can be removed from the base (which you leave in the car) and is sometimes called a bucket seat. This is a convenient way to transport your baby, especially if you have a stroller that can accommodate your car seat. Make sure to measure how much room you have in the back of your car for the seat base.

Some bases are narrower than others, so you want to pick a car seat with a base that fits easily into your vehicle.

A convertible car seat can be money saving because you won't have to buy a new seat as your baby grows. However, one of the drawbacks is that the seat will not detach from the base and cannot be taken out of the car.

Car seats can be installed through the seat belt or your car's LATCH (lower anchors and tethers for children) system. Both ways are considered safe, but do not use both systems at the same time. On forward-facing seats, you should use a top tether to secure the seat. Make an appointment with a certified child passenger safety technician near you to ensure that you have installed your car seat correctly and safely.

Finally, it is best to get a new car seat instead of using a borrowed or secondhand seat, if possible. It's hard to know the history of a used car seat and whether it meets current safety standards or has been recalled. Car seats also have expiration dates. When it comes to the safety of your child, do not take any chances!

Diapers, Bathing, and Other Baby Care

Here are some basics you will likely need for the daily care of your newborn:

- Baby-friendly laundry detergent
- Baby hairbrush
- Baby hats
- Baby monitor

- Baby soap
- Baby wipes
- Bassinet
- Changing pad/table
- Crib
- Diaper cream or ointment
- Diapers
- Emery board
- Fitted crib sheets
- Hooded towels for baby
- Mittens to keep the baby from scratching his or her face (You can use socks for this as well.)
- Nasal saline drops
- Nasal suction bulb
- Newborn bathtub
- Onesies
- Pacifiers
- Socks or booties
- Swaddling blankets
- Thermometer
- Washcloths
- White noise machine

ALL THE OTHER GEAR: WHAT DO YOU ACTUALLY NEED?

There are so many baby products on the market that it can be hard to sort out *needs* versus *wants*. As a new parent, it can sometimes feel like you need every single baby product available because you want the best for your child.

Here are some additional must-have items—and some items that you may want to skip.

Must-Have Items

- Baby carrier (this can help you get things done around the house with your newborn)
- Car window sunshades (so your baby is comfortable and protected in the car)
- Diaper bag
- Humidifier
- Portable play yard
- Stroller (preferably one that can accommodate your car seat)

Items You Can Skip

- Baby shoes (newborns don't walk!)
- Crib bumpers (according to the AAP, crib bumpers pose a risk of suffocation and contribute to an unsafe sleep environment for baby)
- Designer baby clothes (babies grow out of clothes so fast!)
- Diaper pail (if you can take out the trash every day, a diaper pail is not necessary)
- Wipe warmers

Stick with the essentials and remember that baby already has the most important item: your love and attention.

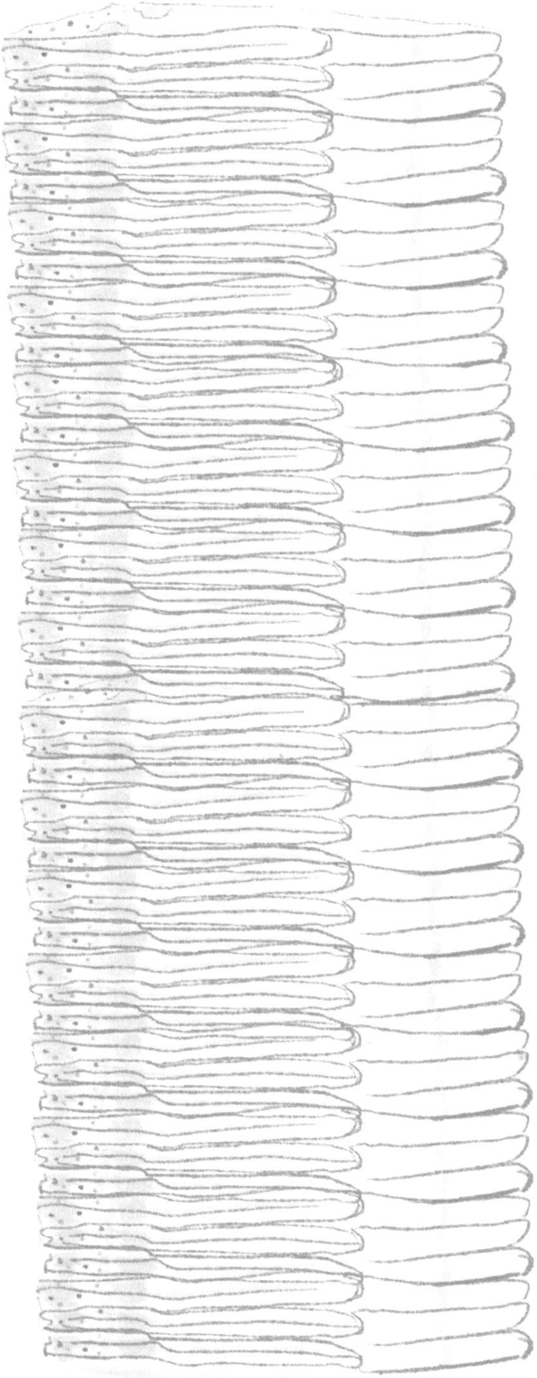

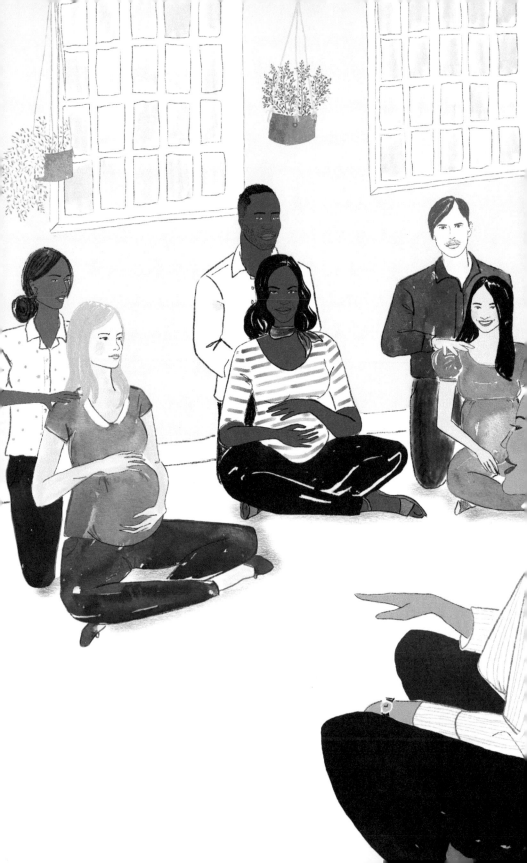

CHAPTER 2

Getting Yourself Baby-Ready

Not only do you have to get your home ready for your baby, you have to start to prepare yourself, mentally and emotionally, for having a newborn. The adventure of parenthood is unpredictable, but there are a few steps you can take to make the transition a little easier, whether you are delivering the baby or not.

Parenting Classes

Being a parent is the most important job you will ever have, so it helps to invest some time into preparing for this milestone in your life. Parenting classes provide tools and strategies for parents to not only take care of their baby but also to be a support for each other.

In a study published in *Maternal and Child Health Journal* in 2015, Dr. Mark Feinberg and his colleagues showed that a series of parenting classes helped reduce parents stress and anxiety and even improved birth outcomes.

In my years of being a pediatrician, I have found that any childhood traumas a parent has experienced can affect the way they interact with their children. It's important to learn how to manage your own stress and address your emotional health and past traumas before your baby arrives.

In parenting, taking care of yourself isn't an option—it's a requirement for being present for your child.

There are a variety of parenting classes available, including CPR for infants, childbirth (if you are delivering), breastfeeding (if you choose to breastfeed), and parenting philosophy classes. You can find information on parenting classes from your pediatrician's office, local community center, hospital, library, and in this day and age, the Internet!

Your Parenting Approach

Before I became a mother, I thought I knew exactly what kind of parent I would be. But motherhood opened up parts of my heart that I did not know existed. The kind of parent I am today is different from the idealistic vision I had before.

There are many different parenting styles and parenting terms that are used today. Here are a few that you may have heard of:

Attachment Parenting. This is a parenting philosophy centered on being continuously close to your child. It promotes on-demand breastfeeding, baby wearing, and responding to a child's cries as soon as possible.

Authoritative Parenting. This is a parenting style in which parents have high standards for their children and use nurturing and positive discipline to help guide them. They communicate frequently with their children and help them meet age-appropriate expectations.

Free-Range Parenting. Parents with this philosophy believe that children become more independent with less adult supervision. Free-range parents let their children solve their own problems.

Authoritarian Parenting. This style is similar to authoritative parenting in that there are high standards for children, but authoritarian parenting often includes the use of harsh and strict discipline. The one-way communication is from parent to child, and this parenting style is not particularly nurturing.

The truth is that there is no manual on how to be a parent. And there is also no such thing as a "parenting expert." You may find that your parenting style changes over the course of years or even in different situations. Your own childhood and experiences will also affect the way you show up as a parent.

None of us are perfect, and kids do not need to see you striving to be the ideal of a perfect parent. They need parents that are nurturing, self-compassionate, and comfortable being good enough parents. This is how children thrive. The real secret to being a great parent is to let go of the idea of trying to be the perfect parent. Understand that we are all simply doing the best that we can.

PARTNERSHIP TIP: CHECK IN ON EACH OTHER'S EXPECTATIONS AS PARENTS

If I am going to be completely honest with you, I need to discuss something no one tells new parents: Your relationship with your partner will change after having a baby.

We are often told that parenthood brings partners closer together, and this is true. But I want you to know that it's also normal to struggle with your relationship after having a child.

Your lifestyle changes from planning weekend adventures to discussing when your baby last pooped. With the list of tasks that you need to accomplish, conversations can become transactional, leading to disconnection and isolation.

As you are establishing your birth plan and plans for breastfeeding, make sure you also plan for how you will maintain your connection with your partner and support each other's needs. It is an important part of being a fully present parent.

Discuss how you will share the responsibilities of parenthood. Make a list of all the tasks you will have when caring for a newborn in addition to accomplishing the regular household duties. Divide the tasks so that both people feel supported. You can also make a plan for nighttime feedings, dividing responsibilities so both partners can get some rest. Plan to revisit this discussion regularly after your baby arrives as needs and expectations can change.

You will spend a lot of time reading fairy tales and happily-ever-after endings to your baby. Most of the time, real life happily-ever-afters require work. But with the right person by your side, the effort is worth it.

Birth Logistics

On the day of delivery, there are going to be many things that will be out of your control. The last thing you'll want is to be figuring out the fastest route to the hospital/birthing center or which entrance to use. Rushing to the hospital unprepared only goes smoothly in the movies!

To minimize stress, it's helpful to take care of some things you can control, such as hospital logistics.

Your OB/GYN or midwife will most likely give you information on how to call the hospital to pre-register. Pre-registration allows the hospital to gather your insurance information and other details so that you can check in easily when you are in labor.

It's also helpful to schedule a tour of the hospital labor and delivery unit so that you'll know exactly what kind of room to expect. In that process, you can figure out the most convenient route to the hospital and the appropriate entrance!

Making Arrangements for Being Home with Your Baby

The Family and Medical Leave Act (FMLA) requires employers to grant time off for parental leave. Assuming you meet the criteria for FMLA, this also applies to partners and adoptive parents. However, employers are not required to pay employees during this leave.

This is unfortunate because not only is adjusting to life with a newborn stressful, it places a financial burden on families.

Applying for leave under the FMLA requires advance notification to your employer and medical certification from your doctor, so start the process early. In addition, research what legislation is in place for your state, because some states offer additional protection for mothers.

Talk to your human resources department and other parents who work at your company. There may be room for negotiation to get some pay during your parental leave.

Finally, if your partner does not get any leave or only receives a minimal amount of days off, keep in mind that being alone all day with a newborn can be overwhelming. As someone who spent most of my maternity leave parenting alone, I regret not reaching out to family and friends for help. Don't be afraid to ask friends and family for what you need. You may be surprised by who comes through for you.

What to Pack in Your Hospital Bag

The best time to start packing your hospital bag is around 35 weeks of gestation when you are close to full-term. If the birth is taking place at the hospital, here are some things you will need for yourself, your partner (if he or she is staying overnight), and your baby:

If You're Giving Birth

- Any entertainment you may want while you are in labor (books, magazines, laptop)
- Any medications you take daily
- Cell phone
- Cell phone charger
- Comfortable socks
- Contacts or glasses (if you need them)

- Hair ties

- Insurance card and ID

- Large maxi pads (You will bleed after giving birth. This is known as *lochia* and will be like a heavy period. The hospital will provide you with some pads, but it's always good to have extra on hand.)

- Nipple cream (if you plan to breastfeed)

- Nursing bras

- Outfit you will go home in

- Pillow

- Postpartum underwear (This is comfortable underwear that's big enough to accommodate the larger pads you will be wearing. Some are even disposable and sit below your belly button to protect the incision if you had a cesarean section.)

- Robe (This was by far one of the best things I packed. You won't want to wear a complete outfit in the hospital. In between breastfeeding and physical exams, a robe is the most convenient thing you can wear. I bought myself a beautiful and comfortable robe to wear in the hospital. It was worth every penny!)

- Slippers

- Toiletries (toothbrush, toothpaste, face wash, deodorant)

- Towel

If Your Partner Is Staying Overnight

- Any daily medications
- Any entertainment for during labor (books, magazine, laptop)
- Cell phone
- Cell phone charger
- Change of clothes
- Contacts or glasses (if necessary)
- Pillow
- Snacks
- Toiletries (toothbrush, toothpaste, face wash, deodorant)

For the Baby

- Bottles (if you are planning to bottle-feed)
- Car seat (Very important! It would be helpful to have it already installed in your car.)
- Onesies/clothes for your baby (Since you don't know how big your baby will be, it may be beneficial to get newborn sizes and larger sizes as well.)

NOTE: Diapers, wipes, and formula are available in the hospital and birthing center, so you do not need to pack them.

Finding a Pediatrician

I've been a pediatrician for more than 10 years, so I know that finding a pediatrician for your child is one of the most important decisions you will make.

You will be taking your baby to the pediatrician every two to three months for checkups during the first year, so it is helpful to do the research early to find the right doctor, instead of switching doctors later.

The best way to start your search is to get referrals from friends, family, and even your other physicians.

Next, decide if you want a pediatrician in a solo practice or a group practice. With a solo-practice pediatrician, you will see the same doctor at every visit. However, if your pediatrician is sick or on vacation, you will have to make other arrangements for your child to be seen. If you choose a group practice, ask if you will be seeing the same pediatrician at most of the visits. Also, get to know the other physicians in the practice since you may see them when your pediatrician is not available.

Speaking of availability, make sure to ask how available the pediatrician is. Not only will you be visiting the office for your baby's regular checkups, but also when your child gets sick. It's important to ask questions such as: Does the office have same-day sick visit appointments? Is the office open after hours or on weekends? Who is on call after hours? With what hospital is the pediatrician affiliated?

Many pediatricians offer prenatal visits so you can meet with them before you make your decision. This is a great opportunity to check out the office and get to know the staff.

You want a pediatrician who takes the time to listen to your concerns and advocates for the physical and emotional well-being of your child. These are qualities found beyond the fancy degrees on the wall.

THE CIRCUMCISION DECISION

If you are having a boy, one of the decisions you will have to make is whether you will circumcise your baby.

Circumcision is a procedure in which some of the skin that covers the tip of the newborn's penis is removed.

The AAP does not universally recommend circumcision for all boys. The decision to circumcise is personal for each family. In the United States, circumcision is usually done because of religious, cultural, or social reasons.

Your pediatrician or obstetrician can discuss the risks and benefits of circumcision with you so that you can make the best decision for your family.

Baby Names

One of the first parenting decisions you will make for your child is to give her a name. Not only will you be saying this name for the rest of your life, it will make up a large part of your child's identity.

States have different deadlines for filing your baby's name. Although you do not need to have settled on a name right after birth, it is easier to fill out the paperwork in the hospital. Making a trip to a government office in between feedings or with your newborn in tow will be more difficult.

As for what to name your baby, don't feel pressured to name your baby according to societal norms, even if you are thinking of giving your child a cultural name or a name that will be considered unusual where you live.

I did not like my own unusual name when I was growing up. But as I grew older, I began to appreciate the origin of my name. I enjoyed telling people that my name was unique and had meaning. I was grateful that my parents did not pick a name just so I would fit in but chose one that kept me connected to my cultural roots.

Pick a name that has meaning for you. It will be the first and one of the most significant gifts you give to your child.

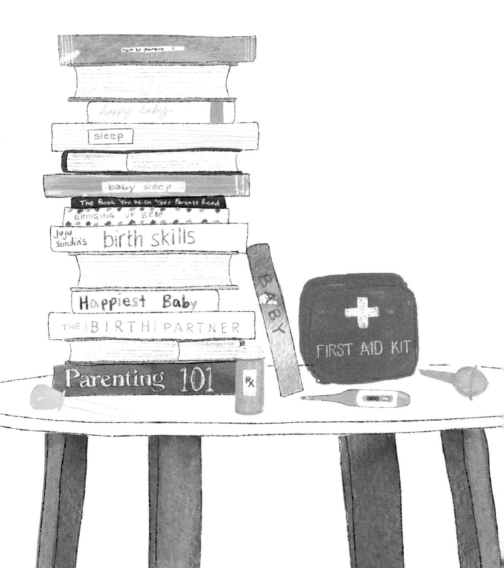

CHAPTER

3

Preparing for Challenging Situations

I hope this chapter does not apply to you. In parenting, we don't want to have to face challenging situations—especially in the very beginning. But it's helpful to be prepared for what could happen, so perhaps this chapter will provide you with a small sense of comfort.

Premature Babies

A premature baby is born before 37 weeks of pregnancy. In general, babies are at a greater risk of complications the earlier they are born.

A premature baby will most likely stay in the hospital for a longer period of time than a full-term baby and will be admitted to the neonatal intensive care unit (NICU).

Premature babies weigh less than full-term babies (who average around 7 pounds) and have very little body fat. Without the extra body fat, the baby is more prone to getting cold so she will be placed in an incubator to keep her warm.

Her respiratory system has also not fully developed, and she may have trouble breathing. To help with this, she may be given oxygen or be placed on a ventilator temporarily.

Not only is your baby's respiratory system still in development, but so is her digestive system. She may initially need some help with feedings through a tube. Breastfeeding may not be possible in the first few days, but you can start pumping your milk to store it for later.

Babies born prematurely will also achieve milestones on a different schedule than full-term babies. But don't worry! Your pediatrician will guide you through what to look for as your child is developing.

Approximately 1 in 10 babies born in the United States are premature, so if this happens to you, know that you aren't alone! Find support from other parents who have had this experience, spend as much time with your baby as possible, and communicate often with the hospital staff. There is strength in sharing your story and empowering yourself with knowledge.

Birth Complications

Childbirth can be unpredictable. And no matter how detailed a birth plan you have for your baby, sometimes life takes over.

Understanding some of the common complications that can occur during delivery will make them easier to discuss with your obstetrician, should you have to face the unexpected.

Here are some common birth complications:

- **Breech presentation.** The ideal delivery position for the baby is head-down. In a breech presentation, the baby presents with their buttocks or feet toward the birth canal. The doctor will usually see the baby's presentation through an ultrasound. They may attempt to manually change your baby's position or elect to do a c-section.

- **Failure to progress.** This is when labor is prolonged and stalls. This could be due to weak contractions, the cervix not dilating, or the baby not descending the birth canal. The obstetrician may give you a medication to boost your contractions, or your baby may be delivered via c-section.

- **Preeclampsia.** This is high blood pressure that is usually diagnosed after 20 weeks of pregnancy. Symptoms can include headaches, blurred vision, nausea, vomiting, and swelling. If your pregnancy is close to full-term, the doctor may proceed to delivery. Otherwise, you may be placed on bed rest or given medications.

- **Umbilical cord prolapse/compression.** The umbilical cord provides blood, oxygen, and nutrients to your baby, but there are situations where the umbilical cord can become blocked. Occasionally, the umbilical cord can protrude out of the cervix (prolapse) or become compressed from the baby's position. The umbilical cord may also wrap around the baby's neck or an extremity. In these cases, the doctor will deliver the baby as soon as possible.

Multiples

Having more than one baby is a blessing for the whole family. But it's also important to be aware of the complications that can arise from a multiples pregnancy.

More than 60 percent of twins are born premature (before 37 weeks of gestation). This number increases with the number of babies a woman is carrying.

Because babies are competing for the same nutrients from the placenta, at some point their growth begins to slow down. They are often born with low birth weights and restricted growth.

When twins share the same placenta, they can develop twin-to-twin transfusion syndrome. This is when blood is diverted from one twin to another through the blood vessels in the placenta. Because of this, one twin gets too much blood, which can affect that twin's heart, while the other twin is a lot smaller. Your doctor will monitor this closely and intervene when necessary.

Most parents are overwhelmed with one baby so the demand of caring for multiples is a lot higher. Make sure you have a good support system in place before the babies arrive. You will need help if one baby is sent home from the hospital before the other. And sometimes you just need a break after back-to-back feedings.

Most important, take a deep breath and know that it will be okay. Despite the exhaustion, one day you'll look back and won't be able to imagine your life unfolding in any other way.

Common Post Birth Conditions

There are some common conditions that can occur in newborns after birth. Understanding what these conditions are may ease your mind if your newborn experiences any of them.

- **Birth injuries.** If labor is long, or delivery has been difficult, sometimes a baby can fracture his clavicle during the birth process. He can also have muscle weakness of the face or arm due to stretching of the nerves. Most of the time, fractures and muscle weakness resolve on their own. The pediatrician will be there to guide you through taking care of any birth injuries.

- **Blocked tear duct.** This condition is also known as nasolacrimal duct stenosis. This occurs when the duct that drains tears from an eye to the nose (nasolacrimal duct) gets blocked. Newborns can be born with a blocked tear duct, which can cause watery eyes or discharge from the eyes. Typically, pediatricians will have parents massage the area between the baby's eyes and nose three times each day. In more than 90 percent of newborns, this condition resolves within a year. If it has not resolved by then, the pediatrician will refer the baby to a specialist.

- **Caput succedaneum.** This swelling of your baby's head can be caused by pressure from the cervix or by vacuum suction or forceps if they were used during delivery. It feels like a bump and usually resolves by itself over a few days.

- **Cradle cap.** This is caused by a buildup of oil and skin cells on the scalp. It can make the skin of the scalp thick, red, and flaky. Pediatricians will likely recommend washing the scalp daily with a mild shampoo or gently brushing the scales on the scalp.

- **Heart murmur.** When the pediatrician listens to your baby's heart in the hospital, he may hear an extra heart sound. This is a heart murmur. About 75 percent of newborns have normal, or "innocent," heart murmurs that resolve on their own. The pediatrician will determine if the baby needs an echocardiogram (an ultrasound of the heart) or if she needs to be referred to a cardiologist.

- **Jaundice.** This yellow discoloration is caused by the buildup of a compound called bilirubin in the baby's blood. Bilirubin is released from blood cells and removed from the bloodstream by the liver. However, because a newborn's liver is immature, bilirubin can build up in the blood. Very high levels of bilirubin can put the baby at risk of complications. Many newborns have a mild case of jaundice that resolves on its own. Sometimes bilirubin builds up to a level that requires treatment. In this case, the baby is placed under special lights that help release the bilirubin from the bloodstream. Jaundice is quite common, affecting 50 percent of newborns. When detected early, it is also treatable, so most hospitals will check newborns for jaundice before they are discharged home.

- **Thrush.** This is an infection of the mouth caused by a fungus that can show up as white patches on the tongue, inner cheeks, and gums. In healthy babies, thrush is not a serious condition and is treated by an antifungal medication prescribed by the pediatrician.

- **Umbilical hernia.** This occurs when the abdominal wall does not completely close during development. There will be a bulge near your baby's belly button; this is a portion of the intestine coming through the abdominal wall. The bulge should be easily reducible, meaning that the bulge should be able to be gently pushed back into the abdomen. About 90 percent of umbilical hernias resolve by the time the child is 4 or 5 years old.

Medical Care in Times of Crisis

While crisis situations, such as natural disasters or pandemics, are rare and unlikely, what they highlight for us as parents is the importance of caring for our own mental health so that we can care for the health and well-being of our children.

A crisis can add a layer of turmoil to new parents' already unpredictable lives. It is even more important in these situations that we embrace the idea of being a good enough parent instead of a perfect one. While maintaining a routine is valuable and can communicate a sense of safety, we also have to learn to embrace the unpredictability of our lives.

During this time, make sure to have regular check-ins with your partner so that you can identify areas in which you can support each other. Enlist the help of your community of friends and family. Crises show us that the best way to get through anything is together, and we should model this for our children.

Finally, if you feel overwhelmed, reach out to a professional for help. There are many ways to connect in person or virtually with a counselor to work through your feelings. A crisis will not last forever, but the coping strategies that you develop to get through it will.

A NOTE ON MILESTONES

As parents, we are often told to track our child's development in terms of milestones, the physical and social skills that a child masters within certain time frames. We also tend to compare our children's milestones with those of their siblings and other children. Most of the time, this causes unnecessary stress and worry.

Milestones are just guidelines. If your child doesn't start walking at exactly 12 months, remember that there is a range of what is considered normal. As you read through the chapters of this book, you will see developmental milestones mentioned, but keep in mind that every baby is different and will develop at a different pace.

This is not to say that babies cannot experience developmental delay—they can. But if you are taking your child to his regular checkups, your pediatrician will monitor his development. If your pediatrician determines that your child has not met certain milestones within the range of normal, many states provide resources, such as early intervention assessments and services.

Finally, remember that every milestone for your baby is also a milestone for you as a parent. It signifies growth and change in your parenting journey. The celebration of your baby's first steps is just as much for you as it is for him.

How to Navigate This Book

Let's face it: As a new parent, or one who is preparing for a new baby, you don't have time to read a book from cover to cover. That's great news, because this is not that kind of book! This book is a resource. Think of it as that friend who always answers your call at 3 a.m. This book will be here for you when you need it.

From this point on, the chapters are laid out chronologically and correspond to the week of the baby's life. Each week will cover what changes you can expect during that period.

Being a new parent is hard enough as it is, and most of the time we don't have the energy to search for answers to our questions. You can always flip to the index at the back of this book (page 137) to find the page you are looking for.

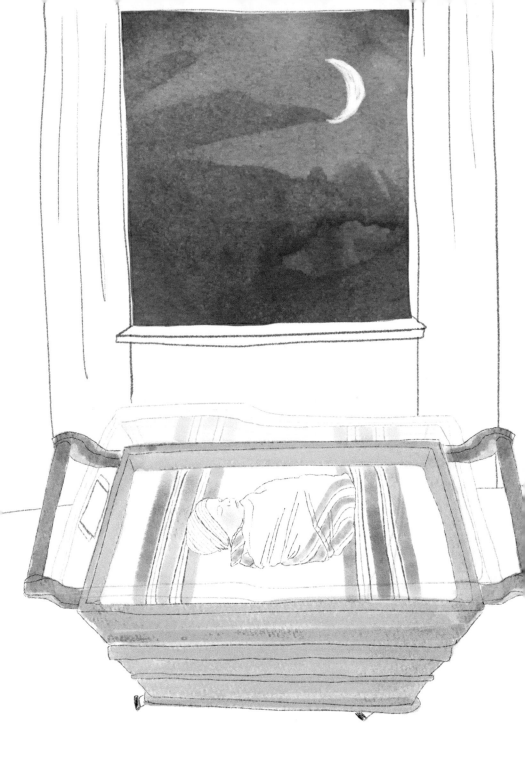

PART TWO

The Baby's Here!

Congratulations! Your baby is finally here! Becoming a parent is one of those pivotal moments that separate your life into "before" and "after." From now on, you will talk about your life relative to this one transformational moment: before you became a parent and after you became a parent.

It is my honor to guide you through the first three months of your baby's life. Each section will cover what typically happens during that week of your baby's life. Remember that each baby is different, so your baby may hit milestones at different times.

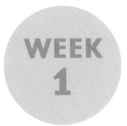

WEEK 1

This section is unique in that we will examine the first two days of your baby's life. Even though the initial days can feel like a blur, a lot happens.

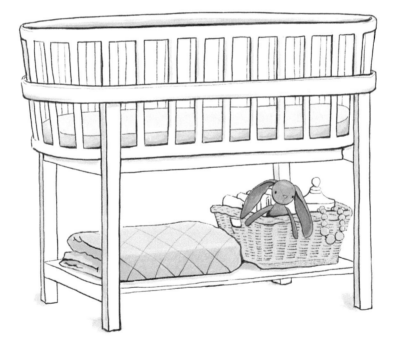

Day 1 of Your Baby's Life

No matter where your baby is born, the first day is all about adjustment. Not only will you be adjusting to the realization that you will now be putting another person's needs first, you will also be learning how to care for those needs.

Standard Post Birth Procedures

There are some routine procedures and tests done during your hospital stay that will help ensure the safety of your newborn. Here are some that you should be aware of:

APGAR TEST

APGAR stands for appearance (skin color), pulse (heart rate), grimace (reflexes), activity (muscle tone), and respiration (breathing effort).

As soon as your baby is born, he will receive an APGAR score. This score is recorded at one minute and five minutes after birth and provides an overall assessment of how your newborn is doing after birth.

Each part of the APGAR score is scored on a scale from 0 to 2. A total APGAR score of 7 or higher means that the initial assessment of your baby is good. If your baby has a score below 7, he may need some additional support with suctioning or oxygen.

This test does not determine your baby's long-term health; it is just used to evaluate your baby in these first moments after birth.

VITAMIN K SHOT

Newborns are born deficient of vitamin K. Because vitamin K is essential for our blood to clot, this can put newborns at risk of bleeding and a life-threatening disease called hemorrhagic disease of the newborn. Therefore, almost all hospitals will give newborns a shot of vitamin K shortly after birth.

ANTIBIOTIC EYE OINTMENT

Most hospitals will also administer an antibiotic eye ointment called erythromycin. This is used to prevent an infection of the eyes caused by bacteria in the birth canal. It also helps prevent against blindness, which can be caused by sexually transmitted infections in the birth canal, such as chlamydia and gonorrhea.

HEARING TEST

Ideally a hearing screen is done before baby leaves the hospital. Between one and three out of every 1,000 newborns born in the United States has a detectable hearing loss. Prompt diagnosis helps babies receive the necessary services that can improve their language development.

JAUNDICE TEST

In chapter 3, we discussed jaundice in detail. Jaundice affects about 50 percent of newborns. It is caused by the buildup of a compound in the baby's blood called bilirubin. Because it is best to treat high levels of bilirubin early, the hospital will do a bilirubin blood test before your baby goes home.

NEWBORN SCREEN

Every state requires that newborns be tested for certain genetic and metabolic conditions. The newborn screen is done via a blood test after the first 24 hours of life. It takes a few weeks for the results, so your pediatrician will follow up on this with you.

Skin-to-Skin Contact

When I was preparing for the delivery of my first child, I remember feeling a sudden sense of anxiety as I thought about those first few moments after birth.

For nine months, my baby had been inside my body where I provided her with warmth and protection. And now, in one moment, she was outside in the world. I can imagine that newborns also feel a sudden unease when they enter this new environment. As such, it makes sense that feeling the warm protection of another person (whether it's mother, father, adoptive parent, or other caregiver) immediately after delivery would make this transition easier for them.

Skin-to-skin contact is when your baby is placed belly-down on your chest immediately after birth. It was first used in 1979 in Bogota, Colombia, where neonatologists Dr. Edgar Rey Sanabria and Dr. Héctor Martínez Gómez were experiencing a shortage of incubators for the sick babies in their neonatal wards. Noting the behavior of kangaroos who hold their babies as soon as they are born, Drs. Rey and Martinez instructed mothers to give their newborns as much skin-to-skin contact as possible. They found that this not only decreased the need for incubators, but also decreased the mortality rate of newborns.

Since then there have been several research studies that have shown that skin-to-skin contact makes breastfeeding easier, increases milk supply, and helps with a newborn's brain development. It promotes bonding with fathers, too, so any parent can experience these beautiful moments of connection with their child.

Baby's First Feeding Schedule

Whether you are breastfeeding or formula-feeding, your baby will need to be fed within the first two hours of life. In the first few days, it can feel like you are feeding your baby all the time because newborns feed every two to three hours. This frequent feeding is crucial for their early growth and development.

Newborns can lose up to 10 percent of their birth weight in the first week of life, but they typically regain that weight by two weeks of age.

While it would be great if all newborns followed an instruction manual, they are human after all, and sometimes they can feed even more often than you expect. The most important thing you can do during this time is to follow your baby's hunger cues. Did you know that crying is a late sign of hunger? Some of the early hunger cues are lip smacking; sucking on the hands, fingers, or tongue; or rooting. Picking up on these early hunger signs instead of waiting until your baby is crying and upset can lead to a more peaceful feeding experience.

If you decide to breastfeed, make sure to meet with lactation consultants at the hospital. They are a valuable resource on how to make breastfeeding easier, more enjoyable, and effective. Take advantage of learning from them when you have the opportunity. If you will supplement with a bottle, read How to Switch from Breastfeeding to Bottle on page 93 for tips on how to bottle-feed.

How to Hold Your Baby

If you have never held a baby before, it is normal to feel nervous the first time you hold your precious newborn. Here are some guidelines for these first special moments. The most important thing to remember is to make sure you support your baby's head. Newborns are born with weak necks and little head control. To prevent any head trauma, always make sure that your baby's head is adequately supported.

When you pick your baby up, place one hand under her head and the other on her back or bottom. When you bring baby toward your chest, you can cradle her and support her head with the curve of your arm. If you place your baby on your chest and shoulder, make sure to support her head with your hand at all times.

Finally, make sure not to bounce your baby vigorously, as their brains are delicate.

How to Diaper Your Newborn

Even if you have never changed a diaper before, you will be an expert by the time your child is toilet trained. Babies go through about 8 to 10 diapers per day, so rest assured you will be changing lots of diapers!

From one diaper-changing expert to a soon-to-be another, one secret I will bestow upon you is to check first if your baby's stool has traveled up his back. This is known as a "blowout." If your baby's onesie has an envelope neck-line, then you can actually pull it down over the shoulders and body instead of over the head to avoid getting poop everywhere. Trust me on this one! If there is no envelope neckline, prepare the bathtub because this diaper change might get messy. You may even decide the onesie isn't worth saving and cut it off instead of removing it over his head.

Now that we have gotten the important information out of the way, let's take a closer look at what you will need to change your baby's diapers:

- **A toy.** If your baby squirms a lot, a distraction is often helpful to keep your baby calm.

- **Changing table or pad.** Make sure to always change your baby on a stable and secure surface.

- **Diaper cream.** If your newborn has a diaper rash, cream is helpful.

- **Diapers.** Make sure you have the right size. Blow-outs often happen because the diaper is too small. There are newborn sizes and larger sizes as well. Have a few diapers handy at every change in case your baby poops in the new diaper just as you are putting it on.

- **Wipes.** Use wipes that are moistened only with water. Wipes with chemicals can be harsh for a newborn's skin. You can also use a water-dampened cloth.

How to change a disposable diaper:

1. Lay your baby on her back on a secure and stable surface. Remember: Never leave your baby unattended, even if she hasn't started rolling over yet.

2. Slide a new diaper under the baby's bottom. If your baby starts to pee or poop in the middle of a diaper change, you already have a fresh diaper ready to catch the mess. Make sure that the side with the diaper tabs is underneath your baby's bottom. Unfasten the diaper that your baby is wearing and lift her bottom by holding on to her ankles or legs.

3. Using the wipes, clean away the stool or urine. If your baby is a girl, wipe from front to back to avoid getting bacteria from stool into the vaginal area. If your baby is a boy, consider covering the penis with a soft cloth in case he pees mid-change.

4. Remove the dirty diaper and place it away from your baby.

5. Apply any diaper creams or ointments.

6. Bring the front of the new diaper up to the baby's belly and fasten the tabs at the waist. If your newborn's umbilical cord is still attached, you should fold the diaper down so it does not irritate that area.

7. Place the used wipes on the dirty diaper and fold it into a bundle using the tabs to fasten it shut. Dispose of the bundle and wash your hands.

The first stool that a newborn produces is known as meconium. It is made up of what your baby ingests in the uterus and can be black, tarry, and very sticky. Between days three and five, the poop starts to transition to normal stool. If your baby is breastfeeding, it can look yellow and like mustard. (You will never look at mustard the same again.) If your baby is formula-feeding, the stool can be yellow, brown, or even green.

How to Swaddle

Swaddling can calm a baby by mimicking the womb and helping your baby feel secure and safe. It also prevents your baby's arms from flailing and startling baby awake (see The Startle Reflex on page 58). Done properly, swaddling is an effective way to calm a fussy baby. While it may seem daunting initially, with practice you will be able to do this quickly.

HOW TO SWADDLE A BABY

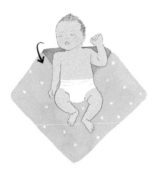

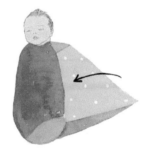

Step 1: Place your blanket on a flat surface. Rotate it to the shape of a diamond. The top corner will be pointed up. Fold this top corner down toward the center of the blanket. Place your baby on her back on the blanket with her head above the edge of the folded corner.

Step 2: Hold your baby's right arm straight by her side and take the right side of the blanket and wrap it over her right arm and chest and tuck it under her left buttock.

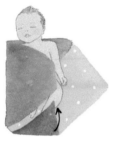

Step 3: Then fold the bottom corner of the blanket up so that it covers the baby's legs, and tuck it under her left shoulder and chin.

Step 4: Hold your baby's left arm straight by her side. Take the left side of the blanket and wrap it over her left arm and chest, and tuck it behind the baby.

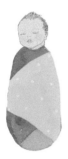

Step 5: Admire your happy, smiling baby!

According to the AAP, if swaddling is done correctly, it follows safe sleep guidelines. Just remember to stop swaddling when your baby starts to roll over (see When to Stop Swaddling on page 103).

WHAT YOUR NEWBORN MIGHT LOOK LIKE

When you first see a newborn baby, don't be surprised if you are shocked. They often look nothing like what you may have seen on TV or in movies.

They can have big cone-shaped heads from trying to squeeze through the birth canal. Their face and eyes can appear swollen, and their hands and feet can look blue initially. They also have thin skin that can be covered with fine hair called lanugo. Most babies are also covered in a white cheesy substance called vernix that helps protect your baby's skin in the womb. Your baby may also have birthmarks in a variety of colors. Most of these birthmarks are benign and fade over time.

Your pediatrician will examine your baby thoroughly after birth. If there is anything to be concerned about, your doctor will guide you.

Don't worry if your newborn doesn't look exactly how you imagined her. Eventually a bright, smiling, adorable baby will light up at the sight of your face. Until then, enjoy these memories while you can.

The World Through Your Newborn's Senses

One of the most common questions parents ask is whether their newborn can see them. Newborns can see about 8 to 12 inches away from their face, which is why your baby may fixate on your face during feeding. It is the perfect distance for them, so enjoy those special moments.

Newborns mostly see in black and white and some shades of gray. Their color vision doesn't develop until about four months of age. They love black-and-white patterns and contrasting designs.

Your newborn has been hearing sounds since their time in the womb. He can be very sensitive to sound and you may notice that he startles easily. He will also recognize the sound of your voice and any other voices he heard before birth.

Newborns have a well-developed sense of smell. He will be able to notice your presence by your scent and, if you're breastfeeding, by the scent of your breast milk. This will make him feel secure, so take every moment to cuddle with your little one!

Day 2 of Your Baby's Life

This is a special day for you and your baby because it is the first full day you will spend together. You will most likely still be in the hospital or birthing center where a lot will continue to happen. At this point you may also have realized that your days of sleeping in and taking naps are over for a while!

Your Baby's First Doctor's Visit

Within 24 hours of your baby's birth, your pediatrician will come to visit and examine your newborn. In chapter 2, we discussed finding a pediatrician and why it's important to pick your pediatrician before your baby is born. If your chosen pediatrician is affiliated with your hospital, they can come to you to do the first newborn exam. Otherwise, a hospital-designated pediatrician will see your baby. This first visit is a great opportunity to begin to build a rapport with your child's doctor.

These are the things the doctor will address during the first exam:

WEIGHT, LENGTH, AND HEAD CIRCUMFERENCE

While newborns lose weight during the first two weeks, the pediatrician will make sure your baby has not lost more than 10 percent of his birth weight. The doctor will also make sure that your baby's length and head circumference are appropriate compared to other newborns.

SKIN

While newborn rashes are fairly common, your pediatrician will check to see if there are any unusual rashes or birthmarks that need further evaluation. They will also check to see if there are any signs of jaundice, or yellowing of the skin.

HEAD

All newborns have "soft spots" in their skull, known as fontanelles, where the baby's skull bones have not yet fused together. There is one in the front known as the anterior fontanelle and one in the back known as the posterior fontanelle. Your pediatrician will make sure these fontanelles are soft and flat and that there are no other concerning areas of the head.

EXTREMITIES

Your doctor will check to see that your baby is moving all of their extremities well.

REFLEXES

Your pediatrician will check to make sure your newborn's reflexes are intact.

UMBILICAL CORD

The umbilical cord and the surrounding skin will be checked to make sure it is clean and dry.

GENITALIA

For boys, the testicles will be checked to make sure they are descended.

EYES

A red reflex test is a screening test to check for abnormalities of the eye. Your doctor will look through an ophthalmoscope to make sure both your baby's eyes have a reflex that is red in color.

FEEDING AND DIAPERING

Your pediatrician will ask many questions about how your baby is feeding, urinating, and stooling. This will help them evaluate your newborn's hydration level. There are many apps that can track your baby's feeding and diaper changes. If you have help with those, they can update the app in real time so you're all on the same page!

If you are planning to breastfeed exclusively, your pediatrician may recommend that you give your baby vitamin D drops daily. Breast milk does not have adequate vitamin D, which is important for healthy bone development.

Vaccines for Newborns

After birth, the first vaccine your newborn will get in the hospital is the hepatitis B vaccine. It is also given at two months of age and six months of age.

At two months of age, your child will get more vaccines. To require fewer shots, some vaccines come as combination vaccines.

Here are the vaccines your newborn will get in the first three months:

- DTaP: diphtheria, tetanus, and acellular pertussis vaccine

- Hib: Haemophilus influenzae type b vaccine

- IPV: inactivated polio virus vaccine

- PCV13: pneumococcal conjugate vaccine

- RV: Rotavirus vaccine

THE COLORS OF YOUR BABY'S POOP

You know you have entered parenthood when texting pictures of your baby's latest poop to your friends and partner becomes normal. Questions about poop are also some of the most frequently asked in the pediatrician's office, so instead of texting an unsuspecting significant other, let's discuss it here.

The first few stools your baby will produce are known as meconium, which is black, tarry, and sticky. It is made up of amniotic fluid, skin cells, and other things that your baby ingested in the womb.

Around the second to fourth day of life, your baby will start to digest breast milk or formula and the stool will start to transition.

If your baby is breastfeeding exclusively, her poop will be yellow in color and speckled with "seeds," like mustard. If your baby is formula-feeding, her poop will be pasty and can be tan, yellow, brown, or even green in color.

If you notice streaks of blood in the stool, if your baby is straining and has hard stools, if the stool looks white or pale, or if there are any other concerning symptoms, call your pediatrician.

How to Handle Visitors

The best advice I can give you about having visitors in the first two months of your newborn's life is to limit them. Your newborn's immune system will still be developing, so you want to avoid exposing them to people who may be carrying an illness, but don't know it since they don't have symptoms.

At the same time, it's hard to tell your baby's great-grandmother that she must wait months to visit!

For those visits that are unavoidable, here are some guidelines that will make your life easier.

1. First, establish a clear time limit before guests arrive. Let visitors know how much time they can stay, and don't feel bad that you need to rest or need time alone to feed your baby.

2. Next, if you have prided yourself in always having a clean and spotless home, come to terms with the fact that those days are gone for a while. Your house will be messy. Take a deep breath and know that this is okay. Don't feel the need to clean up before visitors arrive or the need to entertain. Everyone understands that you have a newborn at home, so it's okay to give yourself some slack.

3. Insist that all visitors wash their hands before touching your baby. It's just good practice, and it's protective for your child.

4. Finally, put your visitors to work! Maybe they can bring you food or help with laundry or watch your baby while you shower for the first time in three days. People feel good when they are being helpful, so let them help you.

The Startle Reflex

The startle reflex, also known as the Moro reflex, is an instinctive response present in newborns from birth. It peaks at one month of age and generally starts to subside by two months of age. In response to being startled, infants tend to flail their arms and legs and jerk suddenly. This can frequently wake them up from sleep, which is one reason swaddling can be beneficial. It is thought that this reflex helps babies stay close to their caregivers and respond to danger such as loud noises or falling. Don't be "startled" when your pediatrician checks for this reflex, because it can alert them to neurological issues.

Days 3 Through 7

Bringing your baby home from a hospital or birthing center is one of the most exciting yet nerve-racking experiences you can have. I distinctly remember sitting in the back of the car on the way home, staring at my baby and watching her breathe!

But no matter how unprepared you feel, in time you will figure this parenting thing out, just like the many parents who have done this before you.

Bringing Your Baby Home

Without the advice and direction of doctors, nurses, and lactation consultants, you may feel a sense of panic being alone with your baby for the first time.

Rest assured that your baby would only have been able to go home if your pediatrician felt that she was doing well medically.

The best advice I was given for that first day at home with a newborn is to have some food already prepared for me. By having packed sandwiches and meals in the refrigerator, I was able to not only feed my baby but easily feed myself as well.

You have probably heard this advice a thousand times already but here it is for the thousand and first time: Sleep when the baby sleeps. It is tempting to do chores when the baby sleeps, but sacrificing your own sleep can make you more irritable, especially in the presence of your baby.

Sleep deprivation can also worsen postpartum depression or anxiety.

Finally, be realistic about the chores you want to accomplish. Your house doesn't have to look spotless; all your laundry doesn't have to get done, and you don't need to clear every dish from the sink. If you have a partner, check in with them to determine which responsibilities you can divide between the two of you. This way both people feel supported and can get some rest.

Just take care of the essentials so you can focus on your most important task: your newborn.

HOW TO LET PEOPLE HELP YOU

One of my biggest regrets after my first daughter was born was not asking for help. I thought I could do it all on my own. More than that, I didn't want to ask others for help because I didn't want to burden them.

What resulted was my being overwhelmed, frustrated, and exhausted—when I should have been enjoying those precious moments with my baby.

In our increasingly isolated society, we tend to forget that back in the day entire villages would help raise children together. Mothers found support in one another's journeys. I encourage you to find your village. During these first few months with your newborn, ask people to help you do the laundry, bring food, or watch your baby so you can sleep.

Not only will you find moments of deep connection with others during a time that can often feel lonely, but you will also feel like a better parent for your child.

Keeping Baby Clean

If the umbilical cord has not yet fallen off, you will be instructed by the pediatrician to give sponge baths only at this time. Use a warm, wet washcloth and wipe your baby's face, ears, and body. Make sure to keep the umbilical area dry.

If your baby had a circumcision, you will want to keep that area clean with a fresh dressing. Wipe away any stool from the penis with every diaper change. You can also use some petroleum jelly on the penis to prevent it from sticking to the dressing or diaper.

Parents often ask how to care for their baby's nails. You will be surprised by how quickly baby nails grow. This can often lead to scratches on their face and body. Parents are generally nervous to cut their newborn's nails for fear of cutting too much. Instead, use a nail file or an emery board. This is a lot easier to manage. Just remember to file your baby's nails when he is calm or sleeping.

What It Means When Your Newborn Loses Weight

During the first week, your baby will lose weight and can lose up to 10 percent of her birth weight. However, during the second week, babies start to regain weight. They are usually back up to their birth weight by the end of the week.

Weight loss in these first few days can cause a lot of anxiety for parents, so it is important that you ensure that your baby feeds every two to three hours during the first two weeks. You should also have an appointment with your pediatrician two to three days after leaving the hospital. Your pediatrician will track your baby's weight and guide you through this period to help ease any concerns that you have.

Tummy Time for Your Newborn

The AAP recommends tummy time for babies beginning on the day they come home from the hospital.

Tummy time consists of placing your baby on his belly two to three times each day for about three to five minutes each time.

Some babies love tummy time, and some hate it. Even if your baby hates tummy time, keep working with your baby because this will help him develop the muscles he'll need to lift his head up and sit. Ideally, this should be done after your baby wakes up from a nap or after a diaper change.

Remember: Never put your baby to sleep on his tummy. This is just for playtime.

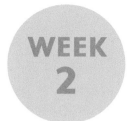

WEEK 2

Your baby is one week old! During this first full week at home, your baby will help you adjust to a new normal of feedings, diaper changes, and intermittent sleep. You will also be experiencing a wide range of emotions, including awe at how your life changed so fast.

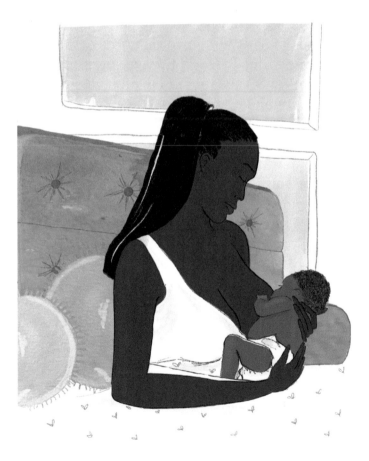

Spitting Up

Almost all babies spit up, but when it's *your* baby who's spitting up, it can feel like you are the only one going through this. It's normal to feel concerned and worried that your baby is not getting enough milk, so let's first talk about why this may be happening.

For newborns, the muscle at the end of the esophagus that allows food into the stomach is not yet fully developed. Because of this, the milk in the stomach can easily come back up. This is known as reflux.

Many babies spit up after they have swallowed a lot of air, such as after feeding or crying. To help ease this, burp your baby halfway through each feeding and again after the feeding. For 30 minutes after feeding, keep her upright at an angle instead of laying her down right away. This will give the milk enough time to travel through the stomach.

Avoid giving your baby more milk after she has spit up. Overfeeding can make spitting up worse.

Your pediatrician will monitor your baby's weight to make sure she is not losing too much. Your pediatrician will also let you know if you should try changing your baby's formula if the spitting up is persistent.

Keep in mind that spitting up is different than vomiting, which is more forceful and can be projectile. If your baby is vomiting after feeding or if there is blood in the vomit or stool, please call your pediatrician.

Your Own Sleeping Schedule

Before I became a mom, I felt confident that I could handle a baby's sleep schedule.When I was a medical resident I worked longer than 24-hour shifts. I was used to staying up all night. *"I got this,"* I thought. What I failed to understand was that after my 24-hour residency shift I had the entire next day to sleep with no responsibilities. We called this our post-call day. There are no post-call days in parenting. No days off. This was one of my biggest realizations during week one.

Your child doesn't care if you haven't slept . . . if you're tired, hungry, or need to pee. Your baby still needs to be fed and taken care of. This is why everyone tells you to sleep when the baby sleeps. As tempted as you may be to finish household chores, use this time to rest, even if it is just to close your eyes for a few minutes.

What to Do When Your Baby Gets Sick

After I became a mother, I understood why every parent in my clinic looked terrified when I told them their baby had a cold. When you have been entrusted to care for a small being whose needs come first, every cough and every sniffle makes you worry.

I want you to know that this is normal. I'm a pediatrician and even I felt a pang of anxiousness every time my newborn sneezed.

Most newborns can sound like they have some mild congestion. Their airways are immature and their nasal passages are tiny, so mucous can build up and make them sound congested. Try using some saline drops and a nasal suction bulb (they usually give you this in the hospital) to clear any mucous from the nasal passages.

Newborns also breathe at a faster rate than adults. However, if you notice your baby's chest pulling in between the ribs (known as retractions) or widening of the nostrils with breathing (known as nasal flaring), call your pediatrician.

The best way to take your newborn's temperature is with a rectal thermometer. Although you can also use an axillary (under the arm) thermometer, the rectal reading is the most accurate.

To take your baby's rectal temperature:

- Clean the end of the thermometer with cool water and soap.

- Put a small amount of petroleum jelly at the end of the thermometer.

- Insert the end of the thermometer about half an inch into the anal opening.

- Wait until you hear the signal to remove the thermometer.

A fever in babies is a temperature of 100.4 degrees Fahrenheit or above. If your baby has a fever, please call your pediatrician's office immediately. There should be a pediatrician on call even after office hours. Because a fever in a newborn can require further investigation, your pediatrician may instruct you to take your baby to the emergency department.

Finally, remember that you have something special called parental instinct. You will know your child best. Anytime you are concerned about your baby because something doesn't seem right, call your pediatrician. Don't second-guess yourself because you are worried that you are overreacting.

You are your child's greatest advocate.

POSTPARTUM DEPRESSION AND ANXIETY

When you are expecting a baby, you are often told about the joy a newborn brings. But did you know how common it is to also feel depressed and anxious during this time in your life? According to the AAP, 50 to 80 percent of mothers can experience the postpartum blues. This can be due to a combination of hormones, fatigue, and lack of sleep.

Ask yourself if you are having trouble sleeping, having crying spells, or feeling ambivalent about parenthood. If so, you may have postpartum blues. The good news is that these symptoms usually resolve within two weeks after childbirth.

If your symptoms are more severe, last longer than two weeks, or you feel crippling worry about your child, you may have postpartum depression or anxiety. If intense sadness or despair is preventing you from being able to do your everyday tasks and care for your baby, I urge you to contact your doctor.

It is important to note that ANY parent can experience postpartum depression or anxiety. The AAP reports that depression in dads is common and can affect 50 percent of dads when the mother also has postpartum depression.

If you or your partner are experiencing any of these symptoms, know that you are not alone. Reach out to your doctor for help. Getting help does not reflect negatively on you as parents. In fact, it makes you even better parents for your child.

How Much Sleep Should My Baby Be Getting?

The first few weeks with a newborn are a roller coaster of sleepless nights. This is because newborns don't have a sense of day and night. Babies do not regulate their sleep cycles until closer to 6 months of age. To a new parent experiencing a lack of sleep, this can feel like an eternity! But do not despair—over time your newborn will start to sleep more at night.

In general, newborns sleep about 16 to 17 hours each day (approximately eight hours at night and eight to nine hours during the day). It may seem like this would leave you with *a lot* of time to sleep, but newborns only sleep in short bursts of 30 minutes to 3 hours. They wake up frequently to feed because their stomachs are so small. In addition, the first two weeks of life are crucial for your newborn to regain her birth weight, so she should not go longer than four hours without eating. Combine this schedule with the tasks of daily living and this can leave you feeling incredibly exhausted!

Most newborns stay awake for about 45 minutes to an hour in between naps. If your baby stays awake too long, it may be harder to put her to sleep because overtired babies become too fussy. Sleep cues such as yawning, staring off into space, and rubbing the eyes can alert you to start putting her down for a nap before she becomes overtired.

Although all parents would love their newborns to follow a schedule, remember that newborns are also human beings who grow and change every day. How often they sleep can vary daily. If you are feeling overwhelmed, reach out to a loved one to watch your baby so you can rest. When you take care of yourself, you are taking care of your newborn, too.

What Your Baby Is Learning

At one week old your baby will be able to see about 8 to 12 inches away. Because she will focus on objects at that distance, she will gaze at you while feeding. This makes those moments extra special!

She will also have a lot of reflexes. She will startle easily to loud noises and will be soothed when she lays on your chest listening to the beat of your heart. She will be learning how to find your breast or a bottle through her sense of smell and her rooting reflex (which allows her to turn her head to start sucking). You may also notice that she lifts her head slightly during tummy time. This will slowly help build her strength.

During week one, you will also come to the realization that watching your child develop and grow into their own person is going to be one of the greatest joys of your life.

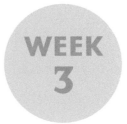

WEEK 3

Welcome to life with a two-week-old newborn! You might even feel like you are getting into a routine at this point. But don't get too comfortable. Over the course of this week, your baby may change his routine—teaching you the true meaning of going with the flow.

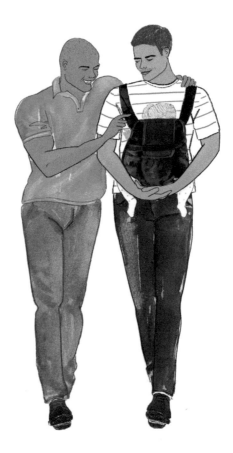

Why Is Your Baby Crying?

Crying is the only way that newborns can communicate. And they communicate often! While it can be alarming to see and hear your baby crying so much, understand that he is just trying to get his needs met.

Most of the time your baby is not in distress. He either needs his diaper changed, wants to be fed, wants to be held, needs to sleep, or feels too hot or too cold. Check to see if your newborn has a hair wrapped around a finger or toe. This is known as a "hair tourniquet"and can cause pain for a newborn and it may be the reason he is crying.

Over time, you will be able to tell what the different cries mean.

Another reason your newborn may be crying is colic. Both of my babies experienced colic, and I will never forget the tears I shed over those endless hours of crying. Colic is when an otherwise healthy baby cries for three hours a day, for more than three days a week, lasting three weeks or more. Babies may also tense their abdominal muscles and bring their legs up to their stomach.

Colic affects one in five babies (and both of mine), so you aren't alone! It is relatively short-lived, lasting 3 to 4 months, but it can feel like forever when you are in the midst of it.

If your baby has any other symptoms such as fever, bloody stools, diarrhea, vomiting, difficulty breathing, or lethargy, please take him to the pediatrician.

How to Soothe Your Fussy Baby

Remember that joy and elation you felt the first time your baby cried in the delivery room? At this point the cries probably trigger significantly less joy as you care for your fussy baby. Don't feel bad; this is completely normal!

In the previous section, we discussed many of the reasons why babies cry. At this time, you may have tried everything, and your baby may continue to cry because, well . . . sometimes they just cry for no reason!

Here are a few ways to soothe a fussy baby:

1. **Wrap your baby.** For nine months, your baby was comforted by the coziness of her mother's womb. It makes sense that she is craving that warm feeling again. This is where swaddling can help. Swaddling can recreate that snug and cozy feeling that your baby had grown accustomed to. Swaddling can also prevent your baby from startling herself and can help soothe her quickly.

2. **Sway with your baby.** In the womb, your baby swayed with the movements of daily living throughout the day. Gently swaying while holding your baby gives her that same safe and secure feeling.

3. **Use white noise.** You may be surprised to learn that newborns don't actually need a quiet environment to sleep. For nine months, she listened to your heart beating, your blood flowing, and other loud noises. A white noise machine (or even an app on your phone) is calming and mimics the sounds of the womb for your baby.

4. **Get outside.** When all else fails, give your baby a change of environment. Sometimes a nice walk around your neighborhood can be soothing for both you and your newborn.

Growth Spurts and Cluster Feeding

Just when you get into something of a routine with your newborn, he goes through a growth spurt! Even though growth spurts only last a few days, they can turn your life upside down.

Your baby will most likely experience a growth spurt between one and three weeks of age. Say goodbye to feeding every 3 hours because your newborn, whether formula or breastfed, may cluster feed, which means that he will want to feed all the time during the day and night. This will also mean that you are even more tired than before and possibly more irritable.

If you are concerned that your baby is not getting enough milk, please call your pediatrician. Reach out for help. Have a friend come and watch your baby, bring you food, or do the laundry. Check out How to Let People Help You on page 60. Most of all, stay patient. Growth spurts should only last a few days, and then you will adjust to a new normal. Think of it as training for the unpredictable ride that is parenthood.

How to Give Your Baby a Bath

Your baby's first bath at home is an important milestone for both you and her. If her umbilical cord stump has not fallen off yet (it usually falls off around two weeks of age), you should continue giving her only sponge baths.

In addition to gathering all the supplies you will need for bathing, ask someone to grab a camera to take pictures. This is one precious moment that you will want to remember!

Newborns shouldn't be bathed every day as it can dry out their skin. Plan on giving your baby a bath every other day. Once you get in a bath time routine, this becomes another great moment to bond with your baby.

Here are the supplies you will need:

- A small cup to scoop water

- Baby lotion

- Baby soap/shampoo

- Infant bathtub (You could also use the sink, but infant bathtubs have an anti-slip surface that allows you to hold your baby safely, which gives many parents peace of mind.)

- Towel

- Washcloths

Giving your baby a bath:

- Bathe your baby in a warm room. Newborns get cold very quickly, so turning up the thermostat a little will help keep her comfortable.

- Fill up the bathtub with warm water only to the point where the bottom half of your baby's body will be covered. The AAP recommends that you adjust your water heater so that it does not go above 120 degrees Fahrenheit. You want the water to be warm but not too hot.

- Next, gently pick up your baby and put her in the bathtub feet first. Remember to support your baby's head at all times. Never walk away from your child while she is in the bathtub.

- Without using soap, dip the washcloth in the water and gently wipe your baby's face.

- Using a mild shampoo or soap, lather your baby's hair with the washcloth. Don't worry about the soft spots on her head (called fontanelles); you can gently use a washcloth over them.

- Using the small cup, scoop up some water and rinse your baby's head. Block your baby's forehead with your hand so that the water does not run into her eyes.

- Using the washcloth, lather the rest of your baby's body with soap and rinse using the cup to scoop water. Remember to wash in between the folds of skin.

- Finally, lift your baby out of the water and wrap her in a towel. Hooded towels allow you to cover the baby's head easily.

- Pat your baby dry. You can then use a hypoallergenic lotion on her body and get her dressed once her skin is dry.

Baby Wearing

Baby wearing is keeping your baby close to you by wearing her in a carrier or sling. To this day, one of my fondest memories of life with a newborn is baby wearing. Because my daughter was calm and awake in her carrier, I was able to interact with her more. She could hear my voice and feel my touch, which strengthened our bond. Not only does baby wearing help soothe a fussy baby because she feels the comfort of your warmth, it allows you to go about your day with your hands free.

Baby wearing also helps develop the same muscles as tummy time. Although it should not be a substitute for tummy time, it is an additional way for your baby to strengthen the muscles of her neck.

There are several types of baby carriers. Here are the most common ones:

- **Wrap.** This is a long piece of fabric you tie around yourself. It creates a snug and cozy pouch in which to place your baby.

- **Ring sling.** This is also a long piece of fabric, but it goes over your shoulder and has two rings at the end. The fabric is threaded through the rings to create a space for your baby.

- **Soft-structured carrier.** This type of carrier has padded straps with buckles. The straps at the bottom buckle around your waist and the fabric pulls up to create a structured space for your baby.

If your baby was premature or in the NICU, check with your pediatrician before using a baby carrier. Always practice safe baby wearing by making sure that the fabric does not cover your baby's face and you can see your baby and easily kiss the top of her head at all times.

PARTNERSHIP TIP: HOW TO SHARE OVERNIGHT FEEDING DUTIES

If you are in a two-partner household, remember that you are a team. One of the first tasks for your team will be to ensure that both members are able to get some sleep. It's no surprise that for humans to function well, they need a basic amount of sleep. It's also no surprise that life with a newborn entails a lack of it.

I encourage you to have a conversation with your partner early on about how you will work together to make sure that both people can get enough sleep to function well as parents. After all, your newborn deserves caregivers who support each other.

If one partner is breastfeeding, the other can help by taking over burping and diaper changing duties. If you are not breastfeeding, you can alternate nighttime duties. If one partner is working a full-time job, you can split nighttime duties between weekdays and weekends.

There are many ways to come to a compromise, and compromise is an integral part of healthy relationships.

What Your Baby Is Learning

Your baby is probably a lot more alert this week than last, and he will look around to notice his new life outside the womb through his senses of touch, smell, hearing, and sight. It's never too early to talk to and read to your baby. Just make sure to get close to his face, as he is still focusing about 8 to 12 inches away. Chances are, he will love these intimate interactions with you!

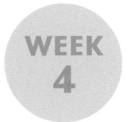

WEEK 4

Can you believe you have almost made it to one month as a parent? Your three-week-old baby is probably much more alert at this point and will require more stimulation. This week we will talk about ways you can play and interact with your baby and how you can care for your own well-being through the power of connection.

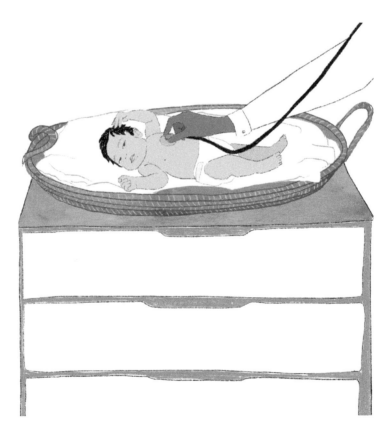

Your Baby's One-Month Checkup

Between two weeks and one month of age, your baby will have an office visit with the pediatrician. If you are in a two-partner household, it would be ideal if both partners attend this visit so that one can care for the baby while the other talks with the pediatrician.

Remember to bring diapers, wipes, and all the supplies you will need for feeding. If you are using a pacifier, bring this as well as it will help soothe your baby while the doctor examines him.

During this visit, your pediatrician will make sure that your baby has regained his birth weight. The pediatrician will also measure his height and head circumference to verify that your baby is growing normally.

If your newborn did not get the hepatitis B vaccine at birth, the doctor will offer the vaccine at this visit.

Finally, you will be asked several questions about your baby's feeding, sleeping, urinating, and stooling. Make sure to bring your own questions as well. Write down your questions ahead of time and write down the doctor's answers. As you have probably figured out by now, being sleep-deprived makes you forget easily!

Parenting Check-In: Get Out of the House!

With your days filled with feedings, diaper changing, and trying to get a basic amount of sleep, you may lose track of time. Weeks can easily go by without you ever leaving the house.

It can feel overwhelming to think about going outside with, or even without, your baby. You may be worried about exposing her to germs or being away from her for too long. But isolating yourself from the outside world is detrimental to your emotional health. Getting out of the house will help you feel connected to the world around you.

Leaving the house with your baby doesn't have to be daunting. Take a simple walk in your neighborhood. This way, you are not exposing her to other people who may be sick, and you get to feel refreshed in the outside air.

It's also important to take time for yourself. Having an adult conversation can make you feel normal again even if it's just at the grocery store or a coffee shop. Better yet, have someone watch your little one and go out for a date night with your partner or a movie night with some friends.

It's taking time for moments like these that make you even stronger as a parent.

How to Play with Your One-Month-Old Baby

Even at this age, it's important to play with your child and respond to his cues. According to research done at the Harvard University Center on the Developing Child, consistent interactions between parent and child help build healthy brain architecture for children. This can affect their physical, mental, and emotional health.

These interactions are known as serve-and-return interactions. It's like a game of ping-pong: the baby serves and the adult returns. For example, if a child looks at you, coos, or even gestures and you respond with a smile or words, these are serve-and-return interactions. Although it may not seem like a newborn can interact very much, as your baby grows and starts becoming more expressive, an environment filled with serve-and-return experiences helps lay the foundation for your child's future development.

Make it a point to interact with your child consistently from the very beginning. Talk, read, sing, and play with him. Even if he is not responding much right now, you are helping to build important connections in his brain. At this age your baby can only see about 8 to 12 inches away, so getting close to his face and making funny expressions— even singing—will help stimulate his visual and auditory development.

His color vision will not be developed until he's four months old, but newborns love black-and-white patterns. During tummy time, you can hold a black-and-white ball next to him. He will turn to look at it, which will help strengthen his neck muscles. To stimulate his sense of touch, you can rub his hand over different items, such as blankets or towels.

This is a fun time to experiment with different ways of interacting with your baby. These moments will help establish a bond between you and your child and will become some of your fondest memories of the new-born period.

READING TO YOUR BABY

You may wonder why you should read aloud to a newborn who doesn't understand the words. Studies have shown that these interactions can help the neural connections in the baby's brain develop. Children who are read to every day from infancy are exposed to more words and have greater language development than other children by the time they start elementary school.

(continued)

Read to your child at least once every day. It's a great idea to make it a part of the bedtime routine early so that it can be consistent throughout childhood.

Start with large black-and-white board books with high-contrast pictures. Books with mirrors or different fabrics can help newborns develop their other senses. You don't need a lot of text in the books because what your baby is listening for is the emotions behind the words.

Eventually, your baby will start responding as you read, and that will make these moments extra special!

How Much Should Your Baby Be Eating?

In general, a one-month-old baby drinks about 3 to 4 ounces of formula every 3 to 4 hours. She will breastfeed about every 3 hours. Each baby is different, so don't be surprised if your baby does not follow this exact schedule.

Your pediatrician will determine how well your baby is eating by monitoring her weight at checkup appointments and making sure that she is urinating and stooling appropriately.

Keep in mind that not all babies will follow an hourly schedule throughout the day, but every baby will develop their own routine or rhythm (for example: eat, diaper change, play, sleep, repeat). Instead of thinking of schedules, think in terms of routines.

Here is a sample routine with approximate times (remember, your baby's schedule may differ):

6 a.m.: wake up, feed, diaper change
7 to 9 a.m.: nap
9 a.m.: feed, diaper change
10 to 10:30 a.m.: playtime
10:30 a.m. to 12 p.m.: nap
12 p.m.: feed, diaper change
12 to 12:30 p.m.: playtime
12:30 to 3:30 p.m.: nap, diaper change
3:30 p.m.: feed, diaper change
4 to 7 p.m.: playtime, nap
7 p.m.: feed, diaper change
7:30 to 9 p.m.: play, bath, bedtime routine
9 p.m.: feed, diaper change, put to sleep
12 a.m.: feed, diaper change, sleep
4 a.m.: feed, diaper change, sleep

What Your Baby Is Learning

At three weeks old your baby's neck muscles are stronger so she will most likely be able to lift her head for a longer period. She may even be able to turn her head, especially if you shake a rattle next to her. As her vision continues to develop, she will be more interested in the world and will start to look around. All she will need is your comforting voice to show her the way!

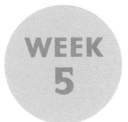

WEEK 5

Your baby is now four weeks old! Remember when I said that milestones aren't just for your baby? Milestones help you celebrate your parenting journey as well, and now is a time to celebrate because you have been a parent for one month!

During this time, you will begin to see glimpses of your baby's personality as she starts to develop into a unique little human.

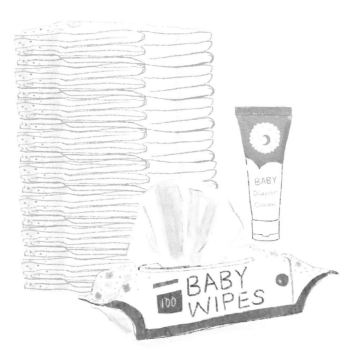

One-Month Milestones

In general, a one-month-old baby should be able to lift his head for a few minutes. He should also be able to turn his head from side to side during tummy time. He will keep his hand in a fist and will be able to bring his hands within range of his eyes. But he will not be able to put his hands into his mouth yet.

He will love looking at your face and will still prefer black-and-white images. He will turn to familiar sounds and startle with loud noises, and, as always, his keen sense of smell will ensure that he can always find his mother's breast milk, if he's being breastfed.

Remember that development can vary from child to child, especially during the newborn period, so don't worry if your baby does not display all these behaviors at this time. However, if you notice that your baby cannot focus on objects, does not startle at loud noises, has difficulty feeding, or has stiff or floppy arms and legs, please talk with your pediatrician.

Tummy Time Part 2

We've already talked about the importance of starting tummy time as soon as your baby comes home from the hospital (see page 62). I hope that you have been able to practice tummy time with your baby over these past few weeks.

To review, tummy time is when you place your baby on her stomach while she's awake for a few minutes each day. Eventually you want to work up to about 30 minutes total per day, spread across multiple sessions.

Not only can tummy time help strengthen the muscles of your baby's neck and back, but it can also help prevent flattening of the back of the head, a condition called plagiocephaly.

There are many ways to do tummy time with your baby. If your baby doesn't like to be on the floor, you can put her on your belly so that she can lift her head to look at you. You can also hold her upright with her head on your shoulder. Make sure to support her neck as she raises her head to turn to you.

Finally, you can make it really fun by placing a bunch of toys on a mat on the floor. Place your baby tummy-down on the mat and lay down on the floor next to her. Laugh with your baby as she looks at all the different toys. Let her feel the joy she brings into your life!

How to Deal with Diaper Rash

Most newborns will have a diaper rash at some point. If you notice red, irritated skin in the diaper area, don't panic!

Most diaper rashes are caused by irritants in your baby's urine or stool. This type of diaper rash is called irritant dermatitis. It can be mild (red or pink patches) to moderate or severe (blistered patches). If your baby is teething or is having diarrhea, the rash can worsen.

There are many steps you can take to prevent and treat a diaper rash. First, change your baby's diaper often. The longer the skin is in contact with urine or stool, the more irritating it is to the skin. Aim to change the diaper about every two hours. If your baby has stool in her diaper, change it as soon as possible.

Use gentle baby wipes and pat the skin lightly when wiping. Use wipes that are moistened only with water and are free from alcohol and scents. You can also use a wash-cloth moistened with water.

Before putting on a new diaper, let your baby's skin air-dry for a bit. This will help soothe her skin. Put a towel or absorbent pad underneath your baby's bottom and use this time to play with her as her skin dries.

Before diapering your baby, layer the skin with a thick paste to protect it from the future contents of the diaper. You can use petroleum-based products or zinc oxide products. These products are thick and may not wipe off completely with each diaper change. There is no need to scrub them off as this can irritate the skin. Just add more paste to what is already there.

If you notice that the rash is persistent or worsening, lasting for longer than five days, is blistering, oozing, or crusting; has lots of red bumps; or is painful for your baby, please call your pediatrician.

MENTAL HEALTH CHECK-IN

One thing I never expected to feel as a mother with a newborn is lonely. I thought being lonely would be impossible when I had another being with me at all times. But the days filled with constant caretaking made me feel disconnected from the outside world.

It's normal not to feel normal right now.

It's normal to feel a sense of loss for the life you had before. It's normal to feel overwhelmed with responsibility. Any parent can feel this way.

First, try to get out of the house. Reconnect with an old friend or find a playgroup and take your child along.

(continued)

Second, ask yourself if your feelings are affecting your ability to care for your newborn or straining your relationship with your partner. It's okay to admit that what you are feeling is a lot to handle on your own. Reach out to your doctor for help. Many parents have done the same.

Remember to give yourself the same advice you would give to a friend experiencing these feelings. Ultimately, the love you give yourself will be the love you give to your baby.

How to Dress Your Baby for the Right Temperature

The simplest guideline for dressing your newborn is to dress your baby in one more layer of clothing than you are wearing.

For cold weather, use layers and make sure you cover your baby with a hat, mittens, and socks. Start with a thin onesie and add a shirt and pants on top. For an extra layer of protection, you can also bring along a blanket.

For hot weather, a single layer of clothing is fine. Most important, protect your baby's skin from the sun. The AAP recommends dressing babies younger than six months in long pants, long-sleeved shirts, and hats that shade the neck when going out in the sun.

For both types of weather, remember that newborns cannot sweat and regulate their temperature like adults, so they are at risk of overheating. You don't want to put on too many layers, even when going outside in cold weather, and you want to take off some of those layers when you come back in.

Eventually, you will figure out what is most comfortable for your baby. Remember to follow your parental instinct. It is a superpower that comes along with caring for a little one!

What Your Baby Is Learning

Your baby's personality is beginning to shine through at this point, and that can be such a joy for a parent. Your newborn is more aware of her arms, legs, hands, and feet. Let her hold onto objects as she discovers her hands. She may focus more on your face. Best of all, she will start to recognize and turn to the sound of your soothing voice, something that will stay with her for a lifetime.

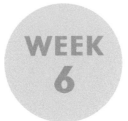

WEEK 6

Your baby is five weeks old! She may be sleeping more at night, which is great because you may be preparing to go back to work soon. If your baby has been exclusively breastfed, this would be a good time to introduce some bottle-feeding to make the transition back to work easier. You may even feel like you have more of a routine at this point. Well, until her next growth spurt. After all, she has to keep you guessing!

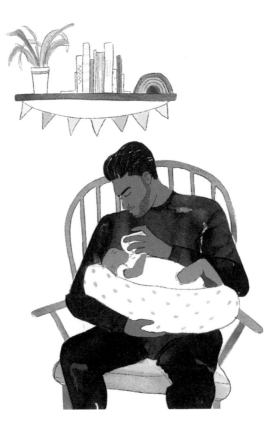

Taking Your Baby Out of the House

By now, you may have already taken your baby out for a walk. After all, both of you need some fresh air! During the first few weeks, your baby's immune system is still developing, so it's good to avoid taking your baby to places with large groups of people until she has had her two-month vaccines.

But life continues to happen regardless of your schedule and sometimes there are events or gatherings you may need to attend. In these cases, ask the advice of your pediatrician before taking your baby out.

You also want to consider the season. For example, taking your baby to crowded places during flu season might not be the best idea. Also, enclosed places with poor ventilation, such as grocery stores or a shopping mall, can increase your baby's exposure to illnesses.

Finally, babies are cute, and everyone wants to touch them! It will be your job as a parent to navigate the delicate balance between yelling "Don't touch my baby!" and being sternly polite. One way to avoid having strangers touch your baby is to wear your baby in a carrier. Strangers are less likely to reach in to grab them when they are snuggled close to you.

If people do touch your baby, make sure they wash their hands first. Don't allow those who have been sick or who have any rashes to get close to your little one. Young children also harbor a lot of germs. Besides siblings, I would caution against other young kids touching or holding your baby.

Finally, if all else fails, just tell people that your pediatrician recommended that no one touch the baby. That's what we're here for!

When Will Your Baby Smile?

The first time my baby smiled at me is a moment that is etched into my heart. After weeks of feeding, diaper changing, tummy time, reading, and playing, when my newborn smiled for the first time, I finally felt seen. And being seen by another human being is a validating feeling.

I can't wait for you to experience this, too.

There are two different smiles that newborns can have. The first smile happens before six weeks of age and is known as a reflex smile. This smile is not intentional. It can occur randomly when your baby is sleeping or even passing gas.

The second type of smile is the social smile. This can happen between 6 and 12 weeks of age and is in direct response to you. You will notice that your baby's facial muscles are also involved in the smile and that your baby focuses on you.

Both smiles are endearing, but the social smile will make your heart smile, too.

PARTNERSHIP TIP: CHECK IN ON EACH OTHER'S PARENT JOURNEY

Speaking from experience, I believe that communication is one of the most important core values in a partnership.

You may not have found it difficult to communicate before you had a baby, but life with a newborn (as I'm sure you are now discovering) makes it more difficult to communicate with your partner. It can be easy to become so preoccupied with the tasks and duties of the day that your relationship becomes secondary.

But here's the truth: Partnership after having a baby is work. You have to prioritize each other, or this central family relationship will suffer.

Carve out 30 minutes each week to check in with each other. You may have to sacrifice some sleep to do it but communicating with each other will help you understand what your partner is feeling. You may discover ways to ease each other's stress, or you may discover feelings you didn't know your partner had.

One thing I know for sure—communication helps you feel seen, heard, and valued in your relationship. And that is worth 30 minutes of sleep.

How to Switch from Breastfeeding to Bottle

If you're a mother who has been exclusively breastfeeding, you may be ready for a break. Whether you want to pump your milk or supplement with formula, it is okay to take care of yourself so that you can take care of your baby.

You may be worried about nipple confusion, which is when babies have difficulty latching back on to the breast after sucking on the bottle. However, the concept of nipple confusion has been widely debated in the medical community. Some believe it is a myth, while others believe it does play a factor in successful breastfeeding. If you want to breastfeed, it is recommended not to introduce the bottle for at least 3 to 4 weeks, until breastfeeding has been established.

What I want you to consider is your emotional health. If you believe that introducing a bottle would give your mind and body a break, then go for it. What matters is that you can be present for your child. Newborn feeding, like much of parenting, is not black or white. You can (and should!) adjust to your changing needs and those of your family.

When you first introduce a bottle to your baby, make sure that he is not starving. It's frustrating to adjust to something new when you are that hungry. Introduce the bottle in between his regular feedings. Also, ask someone else to give the bottle to him. As we discussed earlier, newborns have a great sense of smell, especially for breast milk! Step out of the room, and let your partner take over.

If your baby is resisting the bottle, try different nipple types. The flow of some nipples is faster than others, so you may need some experimentation before finding the right nipple for your baby.

Finally, mimic breastfeeding as much as possible. Instead of pushing the bottle into your baby's mouth, stroke the nipple on the lips and cheeks and allow your baby to bring the nipple into his mouth. Hold the bottle in a horizontal position rather than upside down, so the liquid flows more slowly into the nipple. This is also known as paced bottle-feeding; the feeding is slow, like breastfeeding, and your baby will work harder to drink the milk. You can also use a slow-flow nipple, which will reduce the chances of your baby developing a flow preference and rejecting the breast.

What Your Baby Is Learning

At five weeks, your baby's head control is a lot better now. She will start to lift her head even more during tummy time. She may also start cooing, which is music to every parent's ears! She will also start grasping objects, such as rattles, that you put into her hands. This will make playing with her even more fun!

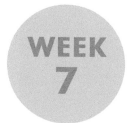

WEEK
7

At six weeks old, your baby is growing fast. He may even go through another growth spurt this week. But his sweet smiles will make the exhaustion and sleep deprivation completely worth it.

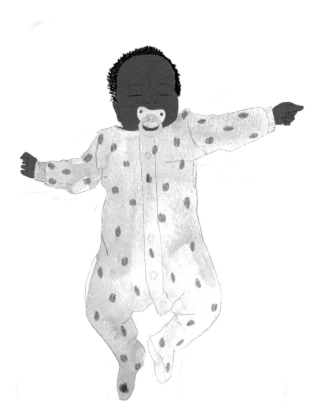

How Much Sleep Should Your Baby Be Getting Now?

By now you may find that your baby has more of a sleeping routine. In general, your baby should be sleeping about 12 to 16 hours per day. He will also take about 3 to 5 naps per day. These daytime naps can vary from about 30 minutes to 4 hours in length.

He will probably also sleep for longer stretches at night, which is a welcome change for any parent! Even better, he will also start to fall asleep faster after nighttime feedings.

Again, remember that every baby is different so if your baby is not following these patterns, there is no need to worry. As much as you can, try to go with the flow of your growing baby. My own babies did not follow these patterns until they got a little older.

At this age, your baby is still too young for sleep training, which we'll talk more about on page 131.

If you are concerned at any point, give your pediatrician a call. It's better to get your questions answered early rather than spending your precious moments worrying.

Is This Normal?

As a parent, you will have lots of questions about your baby. It can be overwhelming to care for a tiny human who changes every day.

To ease some concerns, I've answered a few common questions about what's normal and what's not. Remember that the word "normal" isn't always appropriate because all babies are different and unique in their own ways.

Is green poop normal?

Breastfed babies usually have stool that is mustard-like in color and consistency. Formula-fed babies can have yellow, brown, or even green stool. If you occasionally see green poop in your baby's diaper, there is no cause for concern. If you consistently notice green stool, take your baby to your pediatrician.

Is it normal for my baby's eyes to cross?

Newborns can commonly look cross-eyed. Their eyes are not coordinated enough to always track together until they are about four months of age. Your pediatrician will monitor this development.

Is it normal for my baby to hiccup all the time?

We don't quite know why newborns get hiccups, but they are not a cause for concern. In fact, your baby could have been hiccuping in the womb! Most of the time, babies are not bothered by hiccups and continue to feed and play normally.

Are the white spots on my baby's face normal?

Milia are tiny white spots or bumps on your baby's nose, cheeks, and chin. They can be present at birth or show up a few days afterward. They are caused by dead skin cells that become trapped under the surface of the skin. These spots are common and present in almost half of all newborns. They will go away without treatment in a few weeks to months.

Should Your Baby Have a Pacifier?

This is one of the most common questions I get asked as a pediatrician. Honestly, there is no right or wrong answer. The decision to use a pacifier is a personal one for each family, and no parent should be judged for giving their baby a pacifier. In this section, I'll give you all the information I know about pacifiers and you can decide what will work for you and your baby.

If you are planning to breastfeed exclusively, it is recommended to wait until breastfeeding has been established before introducing a pacifier (about 3 to 4 weeks of age).

According to the AAP, giving your baby a pacifier for naps and at bedtime can help reduce the risk of SIDS. Also, as a mother of two babies who went through colic, I can tell you that giving my babies a pacifier helped save my sanity! Pacifiers can help soothe a fussy baby.

If you decide to use a pacifier, use a one-piece pacifier. Those that are made of two pieces can be a choking hazard. If your baby uses a pacifier to sleep, be prepared for nighttime awakenings when the pacifier falls out and your baby starts to cry. Pacifiers should not be used when your baby is hungry and needs to feed. Finally, make sure you wean your baby off the pacifier by two years of age to prevent long-term dental problems.

Keep in mind that some babies love pacifiers, and some hate them, so your baby may make the decision about pacifier use herself!

Your Baby's Soft Spots

As a new parent, it can be nerve-racking to feel the soft spots on your baby's head. These soft spots are called fontanelles and are areas of your newborn's skull that have not closed yet. There are two of them: one on the top of the head (which is larger) and one on the back (that may be harder to feel).

They make your baby's head flexible so that it can fit through the birth canal. They also give your baby's brain enough room to grow. They are covered by a thick membrane that makes them safe to touch gently. Don't worry! You aren't touching the brain!

The anterior fontanelle (on the top) closes between 12 and 18 months of age, and the posterior fontanelle (on the back) closes at 2 to 3 months of age.

Your pediatrician will monitor the fontanelles at each visit. As long as they aren't bulging out or sunken inward, fontanelles are nothing to worry about.

SLEEPING THROUGH THE NIGHT: IS IT A MYTH?

"Will I ever sleep again?" is one of the most common questions exhausted parents ask me as a pediatrician. And the answer is yes, but probably not through the night without interruptions for a while.

The truth is that once you become a parent, your definition of "sleep through the night" changes. At this point, if you get four to five hours of sleep in a row, you can consider it a win. The next time someone tells you that their baby is sleeping through the night—and you feel bad that yours is not—ask them how many hours that is. You may be surprised by the answer.

(continued)

SLEEPING THROUGH THE NIGHT: IS IT A MYTH? *continued*

In general, babies can start sleeping for six- to eight-hour stretches at night between 4 and 6 months of age. But there is a wide range of normal—some babies start sleeping these longer stretches at two months of age and some don't get there until one year.

Every baby is different, with unique needs for growth and development. Just like adults, they have different sleeping patterns. Your baby will get there eventually. And one day you will have the opposite problem—a teenager who sleeps too much!

What Your Baby Is Learning

At six weeks of age your baby will spend more time marveling at your face, and she will turn her head toward the sound of your familiar voice. She will also start to recognize her caretakers and parents. She may also start to track objects or your face as they move. She will be more aware of her hands and feet and may suck on her fist to soothe herself. As you transition your baby out of her newborn clothes this week, it will sink in just how fast she is growing!

WEEK 8

Now your baby is seven weeks old. You may notice that she is more alert during the day and has periods of quiet when she is not fussy. This will be a relief to you as a parent because it will give you a chance to play and interact with her. She may coo and smile back at you, and soon you will develop your own special way of communicating.

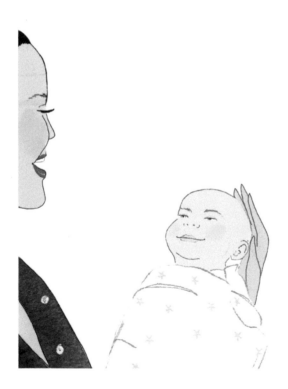

Does Your Baby Recognize You?

Babies recognize their mother's scent and voice soon after birth. With consistent interaction and communication, they start recognizing faces after a few weeks.

At this point, your baby will recognize you and any other caregivers with whom she spends a lot of time. She may smile at you, stare, or make cooing sounds.

Besides talking to your baby right from the womb, make sure all her caregivers spend time talking, reading, and singing to her. This will help her recognize the most important people in her life.

Keeping Your Baby Entertained

Your baby is most likely awake more during the day now and ready to play and explore. In addition to talking and reading to your baby, this is also a great opportunity to play with him.

Because babies love looking at faces, a baby mirror is a fun toy to introduce to your little one. He won't be able to tell that he is looking at his own face right now, but he will probably smile and coo at his new friend in the mirror! It is adorable seeing your baby interact in this way!

While your baby does not have full-color vision yet, laying him down on a playmat with bright, high-contrast hanging toys will provide sensory stimulation. He may even swat at the toys.

Remember that every baby is different, so if your baby gets upset and irritable, he may be overstimulated or just not ready for some activities. Give him a break and try again later.

When to Stop Swaddling

Swaddling is an effective practice to help soothe babies, but it is also not safe to continue when your baby starts to roll over. For some babies this can happen as early as two months of age.

If your baby rolls over when she is swaddled, it can be hard for her to breathe. It's important that you stop swaddling when you notice that your baby is starting to roll over.

Because swaddling was so effective for my babies, I was sad when I couldn't swaddle them anymore. More than that, I was nervous that I wouldn't be able to soothe them. But it turns out that I didn't need to worry so much because they had learned to soothe themselves, which made letting go of swaddling much easier.

PARTNERSHIP TIP: COUPLES THERAPY

In Week 6, we discussed the idea of checking in and communicating as partners on this parenting journey (see the Partnership Tip: Check in on Each Other's Parent Journey on page 92).

If you have been checking in with each other regularly but still feel that something is not right, you may benefit from having a third party help you communicate more effectively. A good therapist will help you see each other's perspective and teach you conflict-resolution techniques.

(continued)

Couples therapy isn't something you should consider as a last-ditch effort. In fact, the earlier you go, the easier it will be to resolve the issues in your partnership. As we have discussed throughout this book, a baby doesn't bring only happiness and joy; this new life change can also strain any relationship.

Going to couples therapy shows that you love, value, and respect your relationship enough to put in the work it needs to thrive and grow. That is the greatest gift you can give your partner and your child.

What Your Baby Is Learning

At seven weeks, your baby will constantly be looking at you, smiling, and cooing. She will be able to see farther away and will start to notice more shades of color. She will love bright, high-contrast objects and toys, and she may even start to swat at overhead hanging toys. Best of all, she may kick with delight when you turn on some soothing music, so gently dance with her—she will love it!

WEEK 9

Here is another parenting milestone to celebrate. Your baby is eight weeks old! You are now officially two months into parenting. The biggest change you may notice this week is that your baby will start to take fewer naps during the day. She wants to be more social now, and that means her personality will really begin to shine!

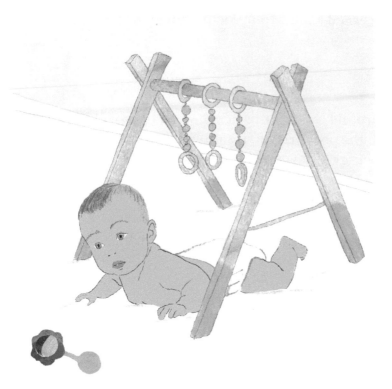

Two-Month Milestones

At two months of age, your baby will be smiling at you and everyone else. He will also recognize your face, and his eyes will follow you as you move. He will coo and turn his head toward your voice. He will have better control of his arms and legs, and his movements will be smoother. When you lay him on his tummy, he will hold his head up and may even begin to push himself up. Best of all, he will soothe himself for brief periods of time by putting his fist in his mouth, which can give you the break that you need!

Remember that every baby will develop at a different pace, so don't panic if your baby isn't doing all these things at exactly two months of age. Your pediatrician will go over your baby's development with you. If there is anything to be concerned about, your doctor will guide you.

Your Baby's Two-Month Checkup

At around two months of age, your baby will have a checkup with the pediatrician. It's probably going to feel like just yesterday that you were in this same office for your baby's two-week or one-month checkup. Time flies when you are sleep-deprived!

Your pediatrician will check your baby's weight, height, and head circumference to make sure he is growing and gaining weight well. The pediatrician will also examine your baby from head to toe.

The doctor will ask you questions about how your baby is sleeping, eating, urinating, and stooling. You will be asked about your baby's development, such as his head control, smiling, and cooing. Don't let these questions stress you out. Remember that babies don't always follow milestones exactly. Your pediatrician will let you know if any further intervention is necessary.

You may also be asked about how you are feeling and coping. You should answer these questions as honestly as you can. Getting some guidance and coping strategies will help not only you but your baby as well.

Finally, at the end of the appointment, your baby will get his two-month vaccines.

Two-Month Vaccinations

While most parents dread this part of the appointment, getting vaccines is harder on parents than children. To help soothe your baby, I recommend having him nurse, feed, or suck on a pacifier during the procedure.

To limit the number of shots, some vaccines come as combination vaccines. Your pediatrician will let you know which vaccines will be given as combinations.

Here are the vaccines your newborn will get in this visit:

- DTaP: diphtheria, tetanus, and acellular pertussis vaccine

- Hib: Haemophilus influenzae type b vaccine

- IPV: inactivated polio virus vaccine

- PCV13: pneumococcal conjugate vaccine

- RV: Rotavirus vaccine

THE CHANGING LANDSCAPE OF MEDICAL CARE

The year 2020 will change the landscape of medicine for generations to come. The coronavirus pandemic has inspired medical providers to think of new and creative ways to deliver medical care to patients. Telemedicine, which had seldom been used prior to the pandemic, has become a crucial part of helping physicians navigate the uncertainty of this pandemic.

Now that insurance companies have started reimbursing physicians for telemedicine visits, physicians and patients are discovering the benefits of connecting virtually. Not only are these visits efficient, they also help patients avoid waiting rooms and offices that can be sources of infection.

It can be overwhelming to become a new parent in these changing times. When you meet with your pediatrician, ask if she offers telemedicine visits. Most pediatricians will want the first several newborn visits to be done in person because they will need to accurately weigh your baby, take growth measurements, and examine your baby for jaundice. But as medical care continues to evolve and innovate, you may find that subsequent visits can be done from the comfort of your own home.

Ask your pediatrician about the office's crisis protocols. Although crises are rare, the coronavirus pandemic has highlighted the need for preparation. Your pediatrician may offer different times for well visits and sick visits or modified hours. Make sure that you will still be able to contact your pediatrician in the event of a crisis.

The year 2020 has changed life for many of us, and it will also be the impetus for change in how medical care is delivered. Medicine will not be the same after this, and I believe it will be for the better.

Daytime Naps

Two-month-old babies usually sleep about 12 to 15 hours per day. This can be split into about 8 hours at night (interrupted) and about 7 hours during the day.

The biggest change that you will notice now is that her daytime sleep will start to be consolidated into two to three naps. Your baby will want to be more social and will be awake for longer stretches during the day. Look out for signs of a sleepy baby, such as irritability or fussiness, so you can put her down for naps before she gets overtired.

As we now know, every baby follows different sleeping patterns, so don't concentrate on schedules so much as routines. Here is a sample routine with approximate times (remember, your baby will show you the routine that works best for her):

6 a.m.: feed
6:30 to 8 a.m.: play
8 a.m.: feed
8:30 a.m.: nap
10 to 11:30 a.m.: play
11:30 a.m.: feed
12 p.m.: nap
2:30 p.m.: feed
3 to 4 p.m.: play
4 p.m.: feed
4:30 p.m.: nap
6 p.m.: play
7 p.m.: feed, bedtime routine
8 p.m.: sleep

HOW TO HELP BABY SLEEP BETTER

Even though babies never stick to a schedule, routines are different. Think of your routine as something that sets the rhythm for a certain time of day. All of us have routines. We can have morning and nighttime routines. When done consistently, our routines communicate a sense of safety for us and help us ease into the next part of our day. This is true for babies as well. Establishing a consistent bedtime routine for your baby conveys a sense of comfort, predictability, and security that can help your baby sleep better.

First, dim the lights in the room to signal that it is time for sleep. Next, turn on some white noise. Your baby has been used to listening to white noise since the womb, so this will likely be soothing for her. Finally, read to your baby or sing a lullaby before you give her the final feeding of the evening.

As your baby grows, the bedtime routine will become one of the most comforting parts of her day, and it will help establish a secure bond between you and your child.

Tummy Time Part 3

At two months old, your baby is probably lifting his head and pushing himself up during tummy time, signaling that his muscles are getting stronger every day.

Your baby can now turn his head and is starting to notice contrasting colors. Use a brightly colored toy or rattle to help him practice turning his head while he does tummy time.

If your baby hates tummy time, do not despair. It isn't unusual. In that case, put him on your chest and talk and sing to him. Make it a special bonding experience!

What Your Baby Is Learning

At two months old, your baby is becoming more social. She wants to be awake for longer periods to interact and play with you. Her brain is rapidly growing and developing with every smile from you. You don't need anything special to help your baby develop, except yourself! Read to her. Talk to her. Sing to her. Do it every chance you get.

Your baby is now nine weeks old! Now that you are a little longer than two months into parenting, you may be ready for a bit more adventure, such as traveling with your little one. Over the course of this week, you will notice your baby becoming even more aware of his surroundings, so it will be exciting to expose him to new experiences. If you want to stay at home and cuddle for a little bit longer, that's okay, too. Not everything in parenting needs to be rushed.

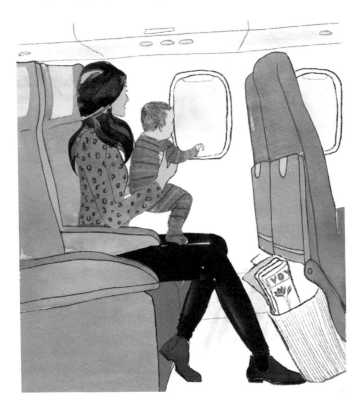

What's in Your Baby's Mouth?

One of the most common infections of the mouth that I see in newborns is thrush. Thrush is caused by a type of yeast called *Candida albicans*. This yeast normally lives in our mouth and genital area, but sometimes it can overgrow. For babies this can show up as white patches on the tongue, insides of the cheeks, and roof of the mouth. Thrush can also show up as a diaper rash.

Many parents can confuse these patches for milk (because milk can stick around as well). But the patches from thrush do not wipe off easily. (Use your finger or a washcloth to try to wipe the patches.) These patches are persistent and do not come and go.

Newborns most commonly pick up thrush through the birth canal. While thrush is typically present in the mouth, it can also show up as a diaper rash. Babies can also transfer thrush to their mother's breast during feeding.

Thrush is not harmful to your baby, but it can be painful and can cause your baby to be irritable. Your pediatrician will treat your baby's thrush with an antifungal medication. If you're a breastfeeding mom and there is thrush on your nipples, this will also need to be treated. Remember to wash and sterilize all bottles, nipples, and pacifiers.

With an irritable baby who is having difficulty feeding, thrush can be stressful for you as a parent. But with the right treatment, it is usually short-lived, and your baby will be back to herself very soon!

TRAVELING WITH YOUR BABY

Before I had a child, everyone would tell me to take fun trips before I had children because traveling would all end when baby came along. It turns out that my oldest daughter had taken more flights before she turned two than my husband had taken in his entire life!

You can travel with a baby. There are just some considerations you must keep in mind.

First, try not to travel during flu season or to places where there is an outbreak of an illness. Your newborn is too young for some vaccines, such as for the flu and measles, so it may not make sense to take the risk of exposure.

Next, evaluate the safety of your destination. You don't want to go somewhere, like a remote island, where medical care or formula would be difficult to obtain if you need it. This is also a risk not worth taking.

If you are flying, try to get a separate seat for your baby, if possible. While the Federal Aviation Administration does not require that you buy a seat for a baby younger than two years of age, turbulence can make it hard to protect a baby who is sitting in your lap. You can take a car seat that has been approved for air travel for extra comfort for your little one.

You may also want to fly during nap or sleep times. The first red-eye flight I ever took was with my baby—and because it coordinated with her sleep time, it was also one of the most peaceful flights I've taken with her.

During takeoff and landing, the changes in cabin pressure can cause ear pain in some babies. To help alleviate this, feed your baby during this time (either by breastfeeding or bottle).

Finally, know that flying with a newborn can be difficult. Despite feeding, naps, and diaper changes, sometimes babies will just cry. Don't let other travelers get to you. Remember that they were once newborns with parents who were just trying to do the best that they could.

Is Screen Time Okay?

According to the AAP, children younger than 18 months should not have any screen time other than video chatting. Although children that age cannot process images on a TV screen, there is evidence that screen use in this age can affect a child's language development, memory, sleep, and attention.

But before you start falling into the endless cycle of guilt about watching an episode of your favorite TV show while breastfeeding, you need to take this recommendation as we should take all recommendations: within reason.

When a parent puts their child in front of a screen or is watching a screen themselves, they aren't interacting with their child. So, watching TV or looking at a screen for 8 hours a day instead of talking, reading, and singing to your child is never recommended. But beating yourself up for taking a 20-minute break to catch up on your favorite show isn't recommended either.

At the end of the day, just do the best you can and remember to give yourself some grace. As they say, "We are all perfect parents until we have kids."

What Your Baby Is Learning

At nine weeks old, your baby's perception of distance starts to improve. This means that she will be looking around and noticing things more. Her hand-eye coordination will also get stronger. She will be even more social and will respond to you with smiles or squeals. Best of all, she will start to appreciate different sounds. Put on different types of music and watch her reaction. Let her play with different rattles. If you can, remember to document these moments with pictures and videos. Despite all the chaos, the memories of these first few weeks will one day warm your heart.

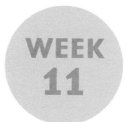

WEEK 11

Your baby is now 10 weeks old! You are probably starting to see more of her personality shine through. She is more active during the day and has a lot to say. Over the course of this week you will start to feel like you are on more of a schedule. And maybe, just maybe, she will start to sleep longer through the night!

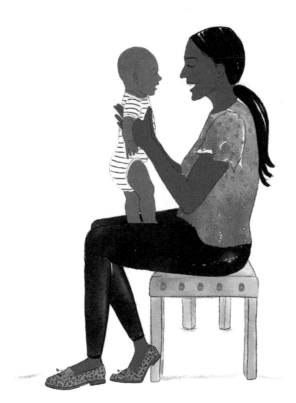

Your Baby's Language Development

So far, your baby has used crying as his main form of communication with you. Sometime between 6 weeks to 3 months of age your baby will start to communicate through a series of sounds such as cooing, gurgling, or sighing. He will not start babbling (combining vowel sounds together, such as a-ba) until 3 months to 6 months of age.

It is fascinating to witness the language development of a baby! It's also rewarding because as a parent you play a large role in this process.

The best thing you can do is to talk and interact with your baby as much as possible. Remember to get close to his face as he cannot see very far just yet. Let him see your facial expressions and hear the different inflections of your voice when you say certain words. This will help him process what words mean.

There are many ways to interact with your little one. I used to narrate different parts of my day to my daughter. For example, I would say, "I'm making dinner now. Do you want some? I'm cutting onions now, and, oh my gosh, my eyes are watering! Don't you hate that about onions?"

It can feel strange to have a monologue, but the more you look at your baby and smile while talking, the more likely it is that every now and then you will get a coo or gurgle in response. And that will make you want to talk even more!

Remember that every child develops at a different pace, so if you have any concerns about your baby's language development, please talk to your pediatrician.

Does Your Baby Dream?

There are two stages of sleep: REM sleep and non-REM sleep. REM (rapid eye movement) sleep is the deep stage during which adults usually dream. Since newborns spend a significant amount time in REM sleep, you may wonder if they dream a lot.

Psychologist David Foulkes, one of the leading experts on pediatric dreaming, found through his research that children do not start to dream until around age two. In fact, for newborns, REM sleep is when the neural connections in their brains are forming and developing. Newborns do not yet have the capacity to imagine. Because of this, your baby is most likely not dreaming at all.

So, while your newborn may not be dreaming about warm and cozy cuddles with you, at least you know that she's not having nightmares!

PARTNERSHIP TIP: DATE NIGHT (OR DAY . . . OR HOUR)

The term *date night* can come with a lot of pressure, and the last thing we need as parents is more pressure!

Throughout this book, I've talked about checking in with your partner regularly. At this point, you may have accepted that the days of spontaneously going to the other end of town or even to another city for date night are gone for a while. But that doesn't mean that you don't crave some time to enjoy each other's company without other responsibilities.

(continued)

As exhausted parents, you may not have the energy to go out for a fancy five-course dinner. And not everyone has the luxury or feels comfortable enough to leave their newborn with a babysitter.

There are many ways to connect without even leaving the house. Make a date with each other during your baby's naptime or when she sleeps at night. You could have a picnic in your backyard or even just enjoy dinner together and watch a movie at home.

The purpose of date night is to reconnect. If you are together, it doesn't really matter where or when it occurs.

The World Through Your 10-Week-Old Baby's Senses

Although your baby is still nearsighted and does not have much depth perception, she will be able to see up to about 8 to 15 inches away. You may notice that she is focusing on you more and recognizing your face. While her hearing was well developed from birth, she will start turning to the sound of your voice and trying to imitate the sounds that she hears. She will also start to show preference for certain textures and feelings. As always, she will keenly recognize your scent—this has always been my favorite part about having young children. For them, you are the center of their universe!

What Your Baby Is Learning

Your baby will be holding his head up even more during tummy time and will push up on his chest. If you hold him in a standing position, he may even bear weight on his legs. He will concentrate more intently on his hands and may even start biting his fingers or sucking on them. You will start to see more of his personality as he shows preferences for different types of sounds; he may become excited by some music but not as excited by other music. Talk, read, sing to, and get to know your precious, growing child!

Can you believe your baby is 11 weeks old already? You are almost past the newborn stage! It may feel like a lifetime ago that you were waiting for your little one to arrive, but soon the next stage of fun will start—when your newborn becomes an infant with a distinct personality that develops more and more every day.

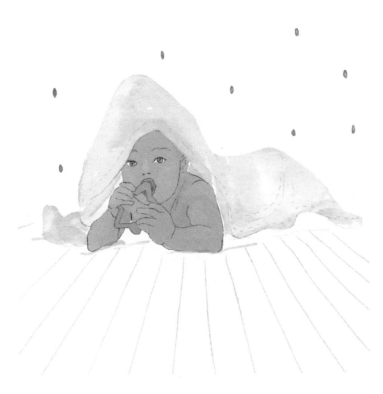

Should Your Baby Drink Water?

Before the age of six months, a healthy baby should not get extra water. They get all their hydration and nutritional needs through breast milk and/or formula. This means that even on a hot day, a baby does not need to drink water.

Giving babies water can fill up their tiny stomachs, making them less hungry for feedings. This can lead to malnourishment and weight loss. This can also decrease a breastfeeding mother's milk supply since the baby won't be feeding as much.

Before six months of age, your baby's kidneys are immature and cannot filter water properly. It is easy to overload babies with water, causing your baby's sodium and electrolyte levels to drop. This is a condition known as water intoxication, which can trigger seizures. That's why it is also not recommended to dilute your baby's formula with extra water.

You can carry around your own water bottle to stay hydrated, but remember that your baby already has everything that she needs!

Keeping Your Baby Safe

At this age, your baby is not crawling or walking yet. But he is wiggling a lot and may even be rolling over, so there are some things to think about to keep your baby safe.

First, always remember to have a hand on him when you are changing his diaper, especially if the changing pad is on an elevated surface. Because babies at this stage squirm a lot, they can fall off surfaces easily. Remember to keep an eye on him at all times. Because he can push himself up during tummy time and grasp at objects, keep hazardous f play. Hide all electrical or appli-

crib, remember to secure those as well.

This is also a good time to start childproofing for the next stage of development. You will want to cover all electrical outlets, pad any sharp furniture edges, and put locks on cabinets in which dangerous household items are stored.

It's only a matter of time before he starts running all over the house!

MENTAL HEALTH CHECK-IN (YES, AGAIN)

You may feel like you are in a routine now and getting more sleep, which can do wonders for your mental well-being. Despite this, something still may not feel right. It is okay to feel this way. It does not make you an unfit or bad parent.

Ask yourself if you are having trouble sleeping, having crying spells, or feeling ambivalent about parenthood. You may feel crippling worry about your child or feel an overwhelming sense of sadness.

The first step is to acknowledge your feelings. You may also want to share them with your partner. The next step is to contact your doctor so you can get the help that you deserve.

If spraining your ankle would cause you to go to the emergency room, then this emotional pain you are feeling deserves the same amount of urgency and care. Learning to care for your mental health the same way you would care for your physical health is what you must model for your children.

What Your Baby Is Learning

Now that your little one is obsessed with her hands, it's a great time to start playing games such as peekaboo with her. You can also put her hands together as if to clap them. She may also start using both of her hands to grasp a toy. She will also start to put everything in her mouth, so remember to keep smaller objects that she could swallow away from her reach.

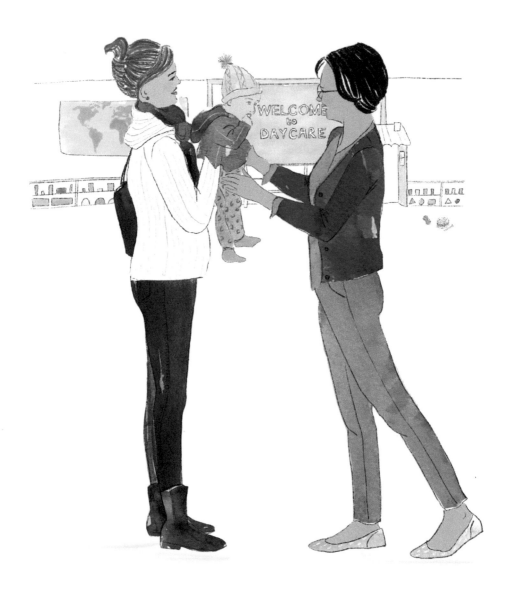

Beyond
Three Months

You are now officially the parent of a three-month-old infant. This is one of the most significant parenting milestones you will celebrate. You have passed the newborn stage!

One of the biggest things I want you to take away from these last three months is this: Parenting occurs in phases, and phases pass. Remember this especially in those hard times when you are wondering how you will possibly take care of this little human. But also remember this in the happy moments so you take every opportunity to savor time with your little one.

But most of all, know that you have survived and thrived through this phase and will continue to do so beyond this age and this book.

Three-Month Milestones

At three months, your baby has graduated from newborn to infant. Along with this, she will also start to lose a lot of her newborn reflexes. She will have much greater control of her arms and legs and will have smoother movements. She will kick her legs when she is lying on her back and bring her hands to her mouth to suck on her fingers and thumbs.

During tummy time, she will lift her head and chest. She may also start grasping at objects and shaking rattles. When you put her in the standing position, she will bear weight on her legs.

She will be more communicative and may imitate some sounds. She will follow objects as they move around the room. She will coo, sigh, and may even begin to babble! Best of all, she will start to recognize you and other caregivers.

Remember that every baby will hit milestones at different times. It's more important to see the bigger picture—your baby is becoming more social and more aware of her surroundings. Soon she will show you all the nuances of her delightful personality!

Going Back to Work

I have to be honest. After almost three months of being at home with my baby, I was itching to go back to work. I loved my daughter, of course, but I also craved adult conversations during the day. I wanted to think about something other than the next diaper.

I thought the transition back to work would be easy.

When I sat in my car and cried for 30 minutes after dropping off my daughter at day care, however, I discovered it would be harder than I thought.

The great poet Rumi said, "Life is a balance between holding on and letting go." And so is parenthood.

Part of me wanted to run back into the day care, take my daughter home, and forget about working altogether. But the other part of me knew that this was one of the first emotional challenges I would have to cross as a parent: I needed to learn to let go so that both she and I could grow.

For my daughter, my transition back to work was easier because I had started to let other people feed her with the bottle about two weeks before I went back to work. This way, she had gotten used to other caregivers. I also did a trial run at the day care for a few hours and let her get to know the environment and the care providers. This made such a big difference!

For the first few weeks, the day care staff sent me pictures of my daughter during the day and I called regularly to check in. This helped alleviate the incredible amount of guilt I was feeling.

The hardest part about going back to work will be learning to manage your own emotions. You will have to learn to let go and you will likely feel guilty about doing so. No wonder everyone talks about parental guilt! It's a part of being a parent, and it means that you love and care for your child.

While this emotion won't magically disappear, the next time guilt comes around, take a step back and give yourself the advice you would give to a good friend: You are doing your best. You are enough. And both you and your child will learn to adjust and thrive.

Childcare Options

The best advice I can give you about childcare options for your baby is to start early and get referrals from other parents. Some day cares have long wait times (my daughter's day care had a wait time of almost one year!) and you will want to take the time to find the right caregiver for your child. Make sure the day care you are considering is licensed and has passed all state and local inspections.

The benefit of choosing a day-care facility (over a single private caregiver) is that there are multiple people on staff if someone calls in sick. As a working parent, this was important to me. I also chose a day care that had a curriculum for learning. While I was at work, my daughter was developing important skills necessary for her growth. She was also able to socialize and interact with other kids. However, day cares can be full of germs, so be prepared for your child to get sick a lot initially until she adjusts. This option can be expensive, however, and also may not be flexible enough if you work outside of the 9-to-5 workday.

A more flexible option is a nanny or an au pair (a nanny who lives with you). The right nanny or au pair can develop a strong bond with your child and family. He or she can also help with other tasks around the house and work flexible hours to cover weekends and evenings. But you will need to have a backup plan for when your nanny is sick, on vacation, or, in the worst-case scenario, quits. Furthermore, this option can be expensive, and it will be your responsibility to do all the background checks and verify references before you bring a new person into your home.

The needs of every family are different, so there is no right or wrong option for your child. Do your research and pick an option that works best for your family's current needs at this time. Remember that life has seasons, and seasons change.

What works now may not work well later. Keep an open mind and learn to adjust to the needs of your growing child!

SLEEP TRAINING

Sleep training is when you teach your baby to fall asleep and stay asleep without help from you. Although this is not an idea every parent believes in, I can understand why some parents want to sleep train their child.

As you start to think about the transition back to work, or just crave more sleep after months of sleep deprivation, you might consider the idea of sleep training. In general, sleep training is not recommended until your infant is about 4 to 6 months of age. You want your baby to be able to self-soothe and go without feedings through the night. However, some parents have successfully sleep trained their babies at three months of age and some pediatricians recommend early sleep training. Discuss with your pediatrician the best time to start sleep training your baby.

One of the biggest misconceptions of sleep training is just letting your baby "cry it out" (which is one method of sleep training in which you let your baby cry until she falls asleep without any intervention from you). In fact, there many ways to sleep train your child, including some that are much gentler than "crying it out." Do some research to find a method that works for you and your baby.

If you have a partner, you'll need your partner to be on the same page as you when it comes to sleep training. Sleep training is a commitment, and both partners will have to participate for it to work.

(continued)

SLEEP TRAINING *continued*

Also, don't expect that once you sleep train your child, he will fall asleep like clockwork and stay asleep every night. As you will soon learn, sleep regressions do happen, and sleep schedules can change.

Finally, don't judge other parents for their choices. There is no evidence that shows either sleep training or not harms or benefits a child in the long-term.

Do what works best for your family!

Looking Ahead: Four to Twelve Months

As you continue this journey, you'll have so many more milestones to celebrate. These include sitting up (between 6 and 9 months), crawling (between 9 and 12 months), your baby's first steps (between 9 and 12 months), and your baby's first words (toward the end of the year).

Remember that every baby is different and will achieve milestones at different times. Your pediatrician will let you know if intervention is needed. There are many resources and assessment services provided by each state, so rest assured that your baby can get any help that may be needed.

As parents, you will celebrate the first time you sleep all the way through the night, the first time you go a whole day without discussing the color of your baby's poop, and the first time your heart lights up when your baby calls you Mama or Dada.

My journey so far in parenting has taught me how love actually works. From the moment my daughters first started walking, I had to learn to let them go and let them fall. But through it all, I always kept one hand on them just to let them know that if they ever need me, I'm right there.

And that's what you have to look forward to: the joy of nurturing another human so he or she can eventually fly, while always providing a safe place for them to land.

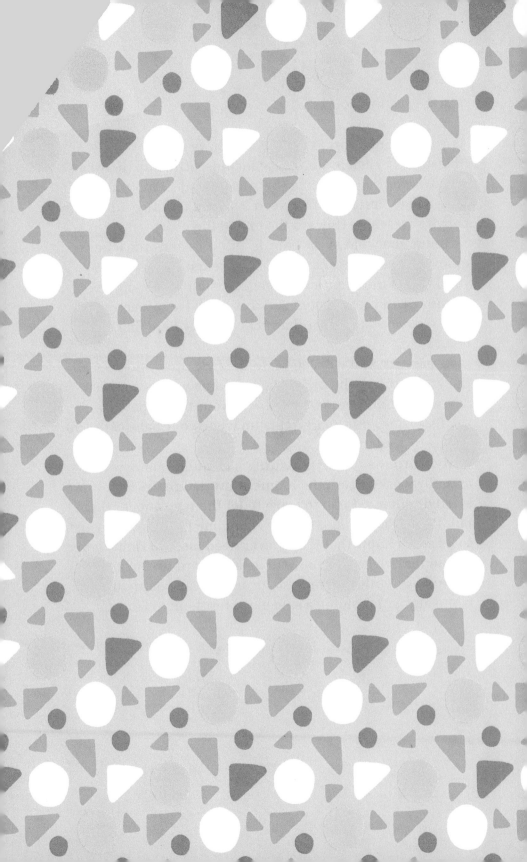

RESOURCES AND REFERENCES

AAP.org is the professional website for the American Academy of Pediatrics. This website contains the latest briefings and recommendations for the nation's largest association of pediatricians.

Feinberg, Mark E., Damon E. Jones, Michael E. Roettger, Michelle L. Hostetler, Kari-Lyn Sakuma, Ian M. Paul, and Deborah B. Ehrenthal. "Preventive Effects on Birth Outcomes: Buffering Impact of Maternal Stress, Depression, and Anxiety." *Maternal and Child Health Journal* 20, no. 1 (January 2015): 56-65. doi: 10.1007/s10995-015-1801-3.

Harvard University Center on the Developing Child (DevelopingChild. Harvard.edu/guide/what-is-early-childhood-development-a-guide-to-the-science) features helpful links about the science behind early childhood development, including videos and articles related to ensuring healthy infant, toddler, and child growth.

HealthyChildren.org is a parenting website endorsed by the American Academy of Pediatrics. On this website, you will find articles on children's health and parenting that can be helpful in the first few months with a newborn and beyond.

Kelly Mom (KellyMom.com) is a website featuring evidence-based information about breastfeeding written and maintained by an international board-certified lactation consultant and mother of three. It is an extensive resource for breastfeeding from infancy and beyond.

La Leche League International (LLLI.org) is an international organization dedicated to providing mother-to-mother support for breastfeeding, including in-person breastfeeding support groups. Meeting locations can be found on their website.

Postpartum Progress (PostpartumProgress.com) is the world's most-read blog on the topic of perinatal mood and anxiety disorders, explaining these conditions in "plain mama English." You can learn about the symptoms of postpartum depression, anxiety, and other mood disorders on their website.

Postpartum Support International (Postpartum.net) is an international organization dedicated to connecting mothers to both peer-to-peer and professional support for perinatal mood and anxiety disorders. Visit their website to find a support group or provider in your area.

Zero to Three (ZeroToThree.org) is dedicated to fostering positive early connections between infants and their caregivers to ensure that babies and children aged zero to three thrive.

INDEX

Skin-to-skin contact, 45–46
Sleeping
  dreaming, 119
  newborns' schedule, 68
  parents' schedule, 64–65
  routines, 96, 109–110
  safety, 10–13
  sleep training, 131–132
  supplies, 4–5
  through the night, 99–100
Smiling, 92
Soft spots, 54–55, 98–99
Spitting up, 64
Startle reflex, 58–59, 69
Sudden infant death syndrome (SIDS),
    11–12
Supplies
  daily care, 14–15
  feeding, 5–8
  gear, 16
  sleeping, 4–5
Swaddling, 50–52, 72, 103

T

Tear ducts, blocked, 35
Temperature-taking, 66

Thrush, 37, 113
Travel, 114–115
Tummy time, 62, 69, 85–86, 110
Twins, 34–35

U

Umbilical cord prolapse/compression,
    33–34
Umbilical hernias, 37

V

Vaccines, 56, 107
Vernix, 52
Visitors, 57–58
Vitamin D, 56
Vitamin K shot, 43

W

Water, 123
Weight loss, 61
Work, returning to, 128–129
Wraps, 76

ACKNOWLEDGMENTS

I want to give thanks to my family for giving me their patience and the time to write this book. To everyone on my publishing team, including the talented editors from whom I have learned so much about this Process. And to all the families I have worked with in my career who have taught me everything about what it means to be a pediatrician and a mother.

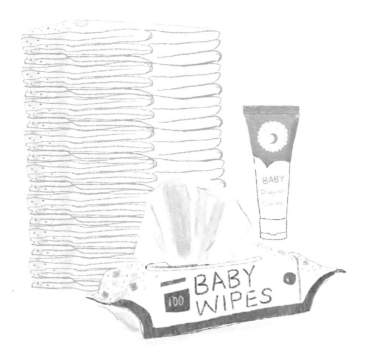

ABOUT THE AUTHOR

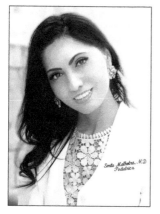

Dr. Smita Malhotra is a mother, pediatrician, writer, and speaker. After completing her pediatric residency and chief residency in New York City, she moved to Los Angeles where she has been caring for children and newborns for more than 10 years. She believes in healing the child and family holistically by combining traditional medicine with alternative therapies, such as mindfulness, meditation, acupuncture, and yoga. She is an advocate for providing children with the tools to cope through the peaks and valleys of their lives and empowering them to take charge of their own health and nutrition. She believes in the power of writing and social media to spread that message and has contributed to the *Washington Post* and other publications.